I0520815

WANT TO GET IN TOUCH?

Email us at:

tlhennig6@gmail.com

or visit us and leave a review:

https://www.amazon.com/~/e/B07TTDHJ8P

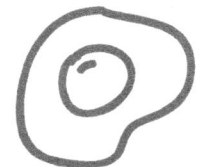 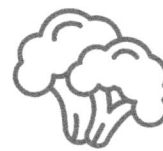 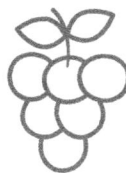 

My name is _____.

My favorite food is

_____.

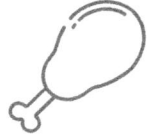

- - - - - - - - - - - -

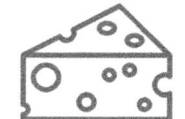

You are growing!
You are strong!
Let's learn about food
to help you along!

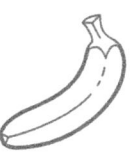 

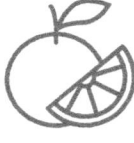 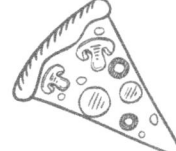 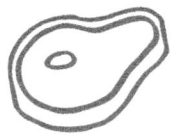

 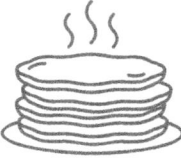 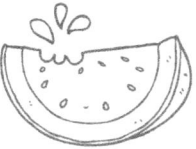

I CAN WRITE

Fruit

I can read and trace

Fruit

Fruit

Fruit

Fruit

Fruit

Fruit

Food is good!
Food helps us grow strong!

Eat Daily:

 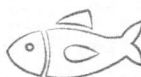

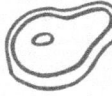 

 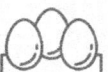

 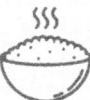

Special Treat:

 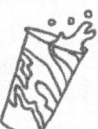

 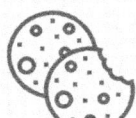

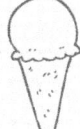 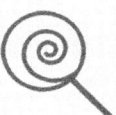

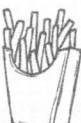 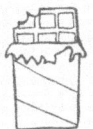

When we make good choices, we can't go wrong!

I CAN WRITE
Vegetable
I can read and trace

Vegetable

Vegetable

Vegetable

Vegetable

Vegetable

Vegetable

Name: _____   Date: _____

Food Scramble

Unscramble the letters, write the word down
and connect to the correct **Food** element

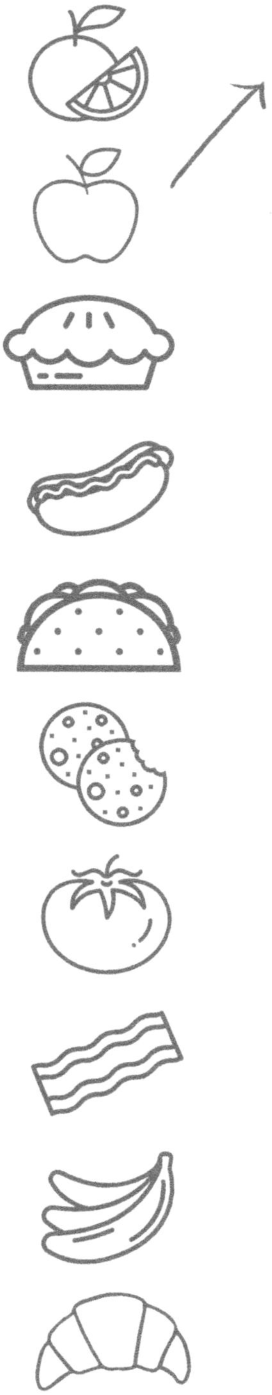

PEAPL	APPLE
OACT	
AMTOTO	
SACNTRSIO	
RGEAON	
AOCNB	
OTOHGD	
IEP	
SBANAAN	
SCOIEKO	

Fruit & Vegetable
Coloring

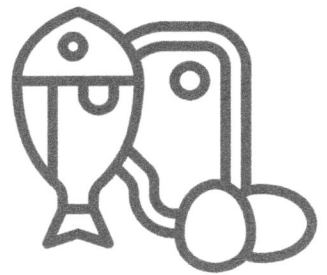

I CAN WRITE

Protein

I can read and trace

Protein

Protein

Protein

Protein

Protein

Protein

My favorite foods

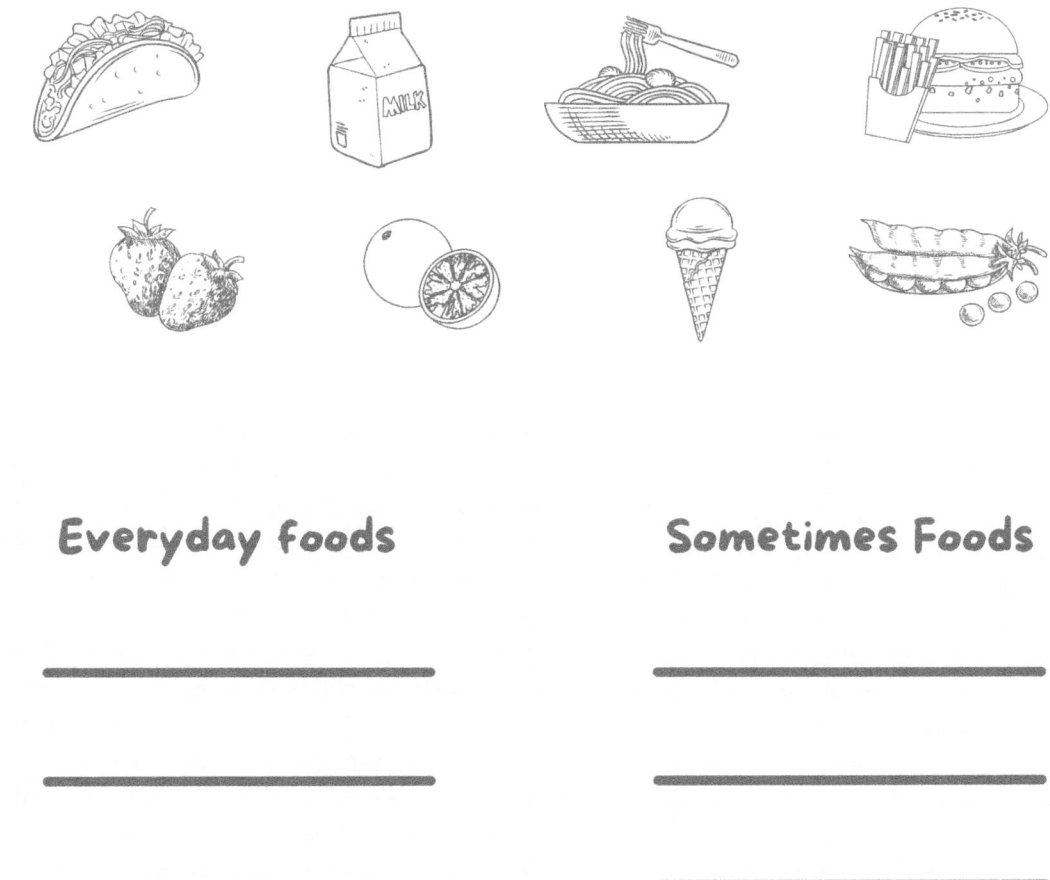

Everyday foods

_____

_____

_____

Sometimes Foods

_____

_____

_____

Everyday foods include the food groups like fruits, vegetables, proteins, dairy, grains and healthy fats. They keep you healthy and strong.

Sometimes foods include sweets, fast food, chips and sugary drinks. They should be special treats and not eaten everyday.

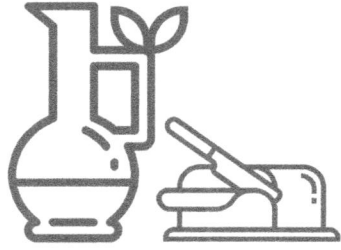

I CAN WRITE
Fats
I can read and trace

Fats

Fats

Fats

Fats

Fats

Fats

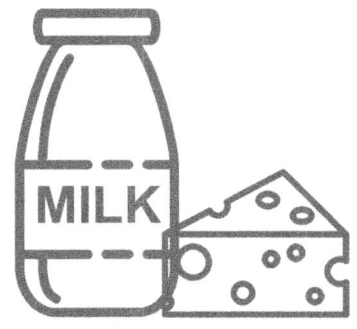

I CAN WRITE

Dairy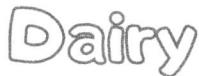

I can read and trace

Dairy

Dairy

Dairy

Dairy

Dairy

Dairy

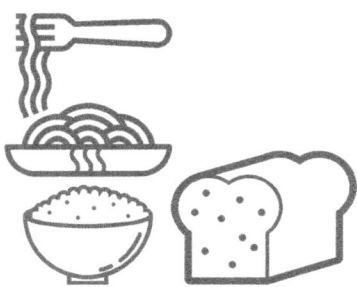

I CAN WRITE
Grains
I can read and trace

Grains

Grains

Grains

Grains

Grains

Grains

Same size

In each group, circle the two
pictures that are the SAME SIZE.

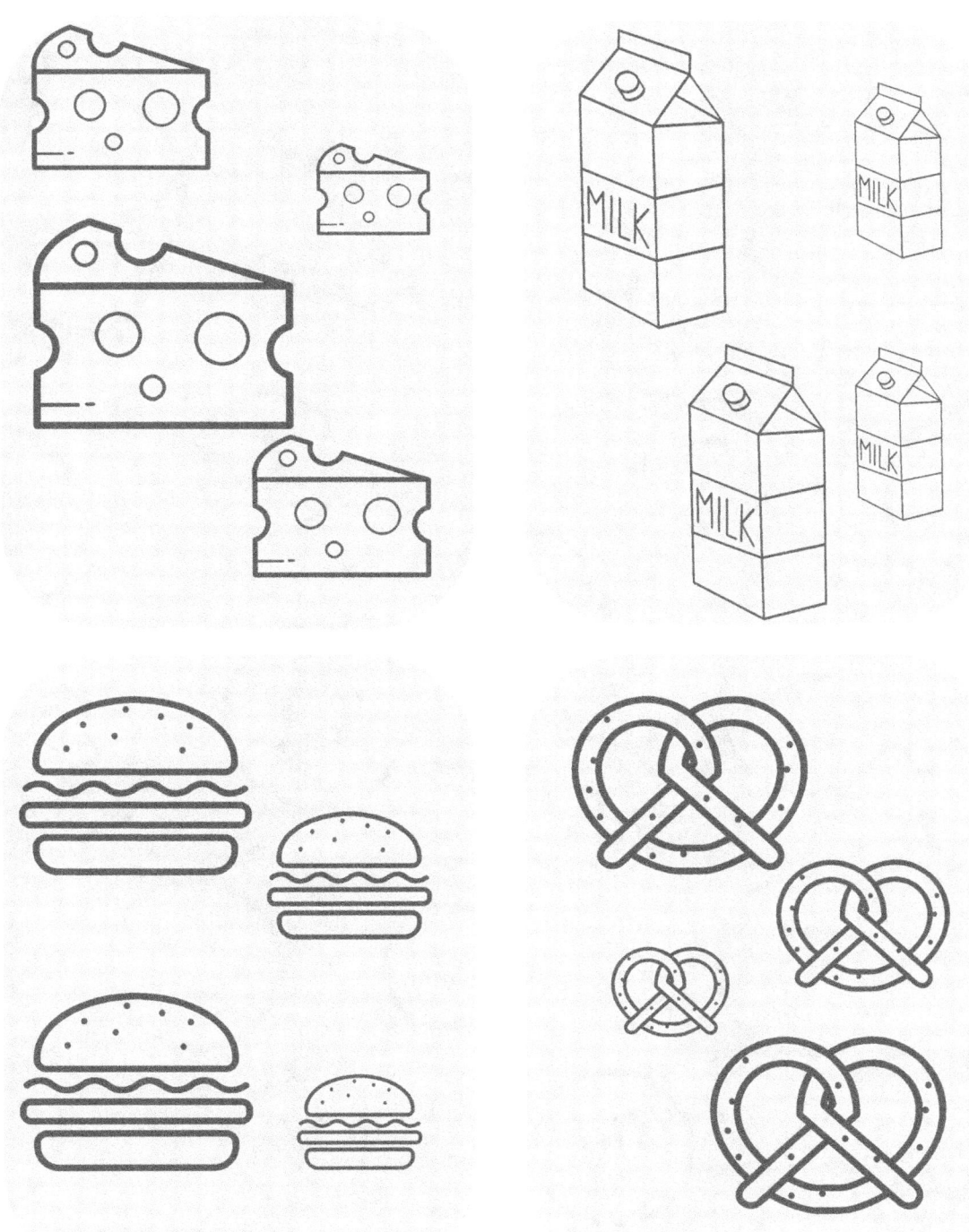

Find the letters.

DIRECTIONS: TRACE THE LETTERS. THEN COLOR THE CIRCLES THAT HAVE THE LETTER YOU TRACED.

is for Apple

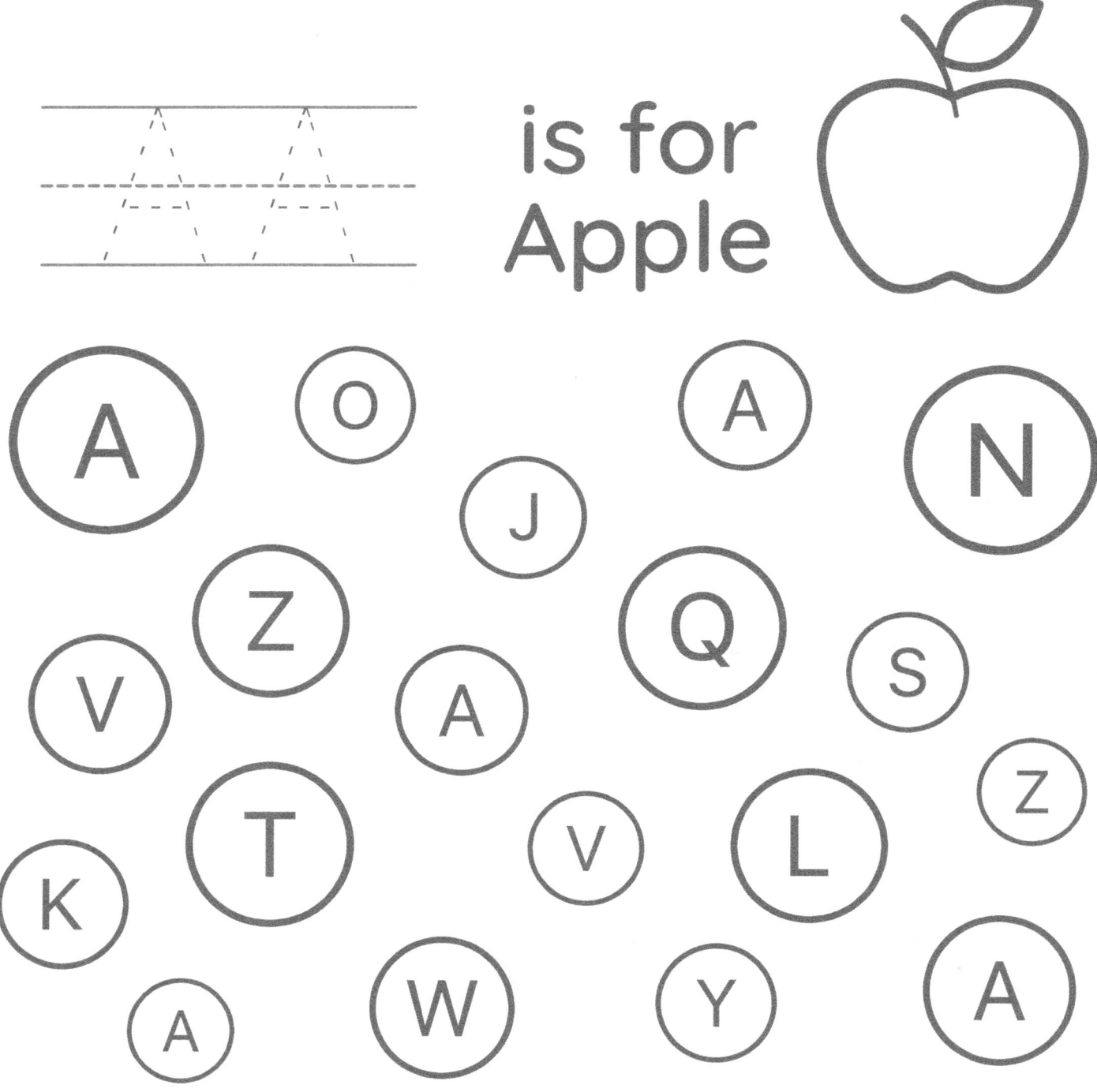

FRUIT

discover, learn & enjoy delicious fruits

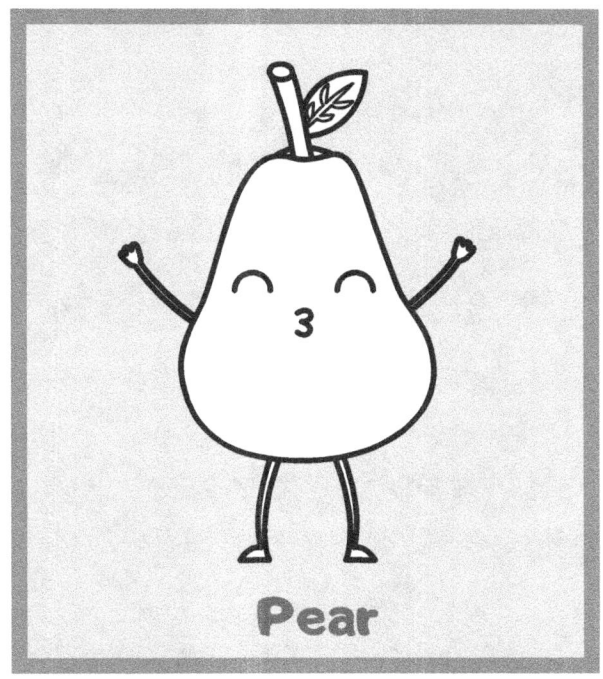

Pear

Fruit is colorful
and fun!

Fruit is a great
snack for
everyone!

My favorite fruit
is:

_____

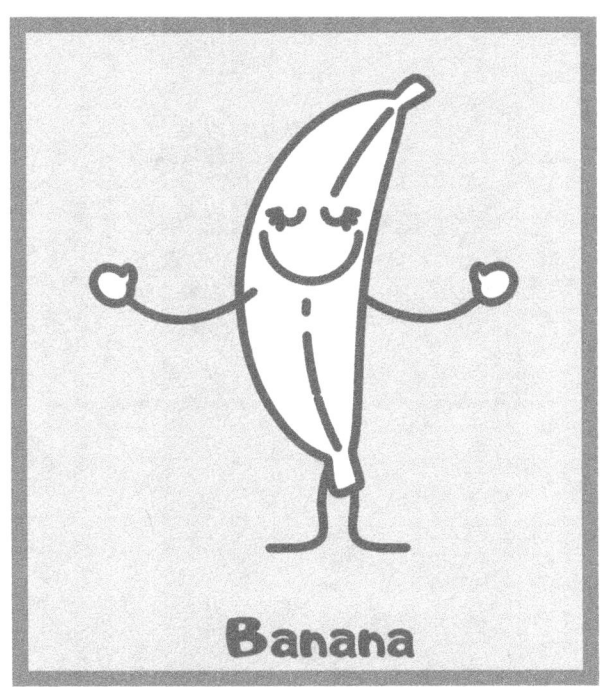

Banana

VEGETABLE

discover, learn & enjoy delicious vegetables

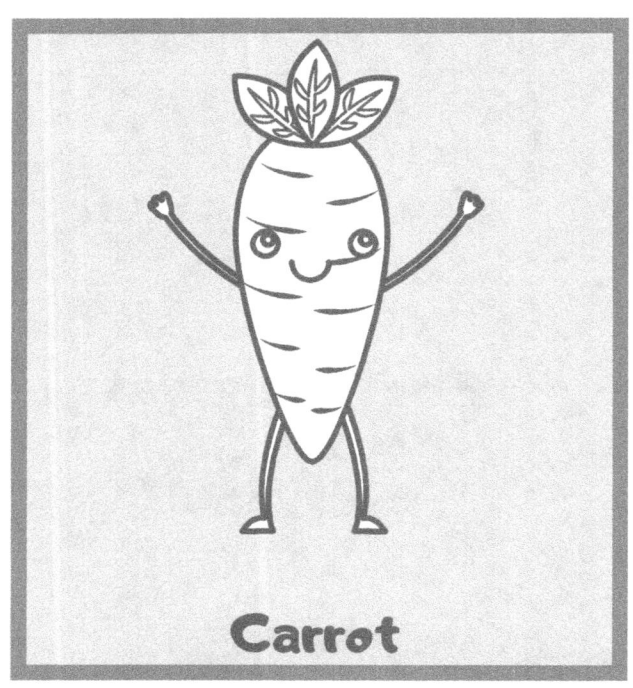

Carrot

Vegetables are packed full of things to keep you healthy and strong!

There are many to choose from, try different colored vegetables all day long!

My favorite vegetable is:

_____

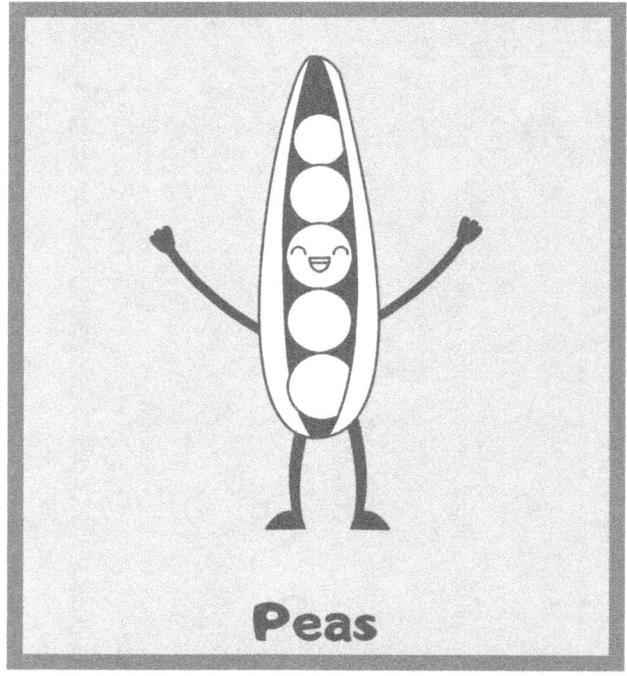

Peas

PROTEIN

discover, learn & enjoy delicious protein foods

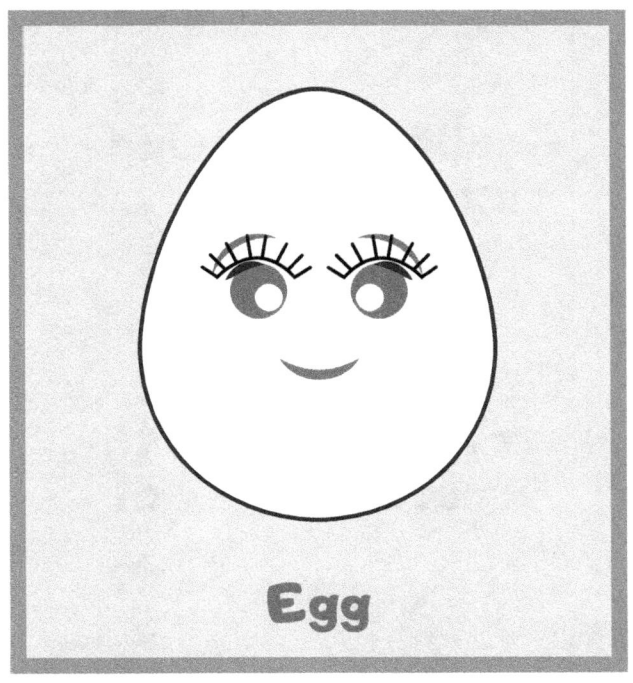

Egg

Protein foods include meat, chicken, eggs, fish and beans.

They help us grow strong and keep our muscles healthy and lean!

My favorite protein food is:

_____

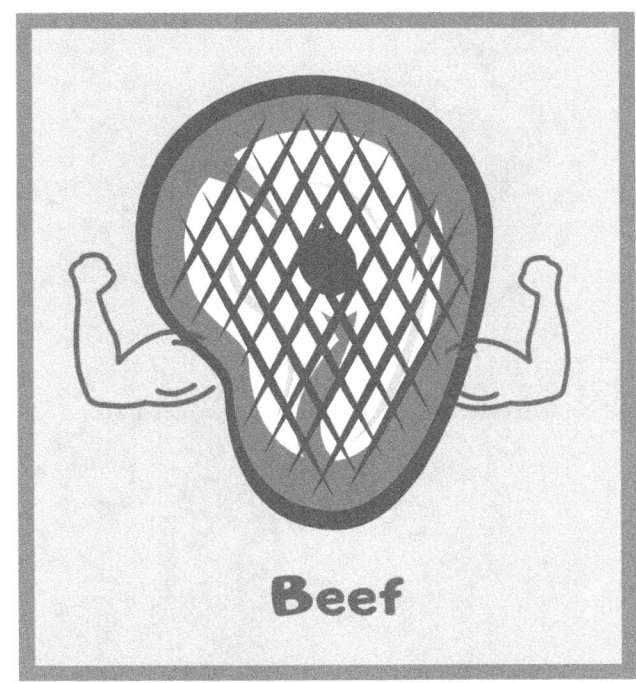

Beef

GRAINS

discover, learn & enjoy delicious grain foods

Pasta

Grain foods include rice, pasta, and all kinds of bread.

They give energy to our muscles and the brain in our head!

My favorite grain food is:

_____

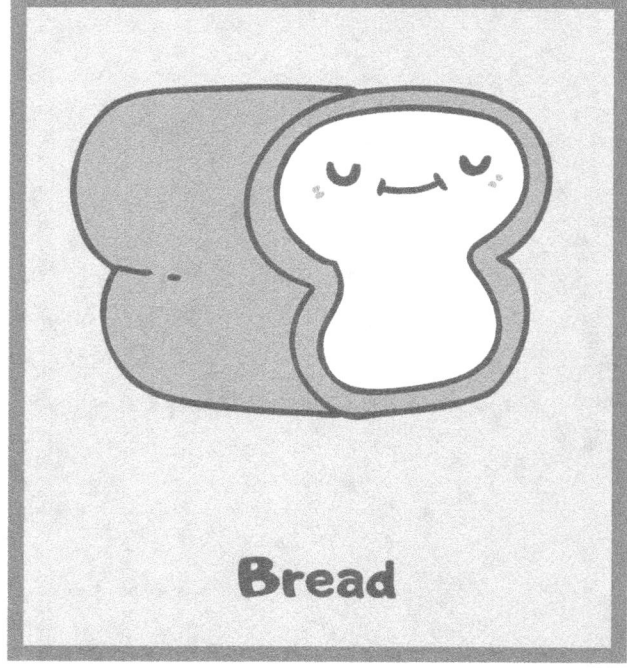

Bread

FATS

discover, learn & enjoy delicious fats

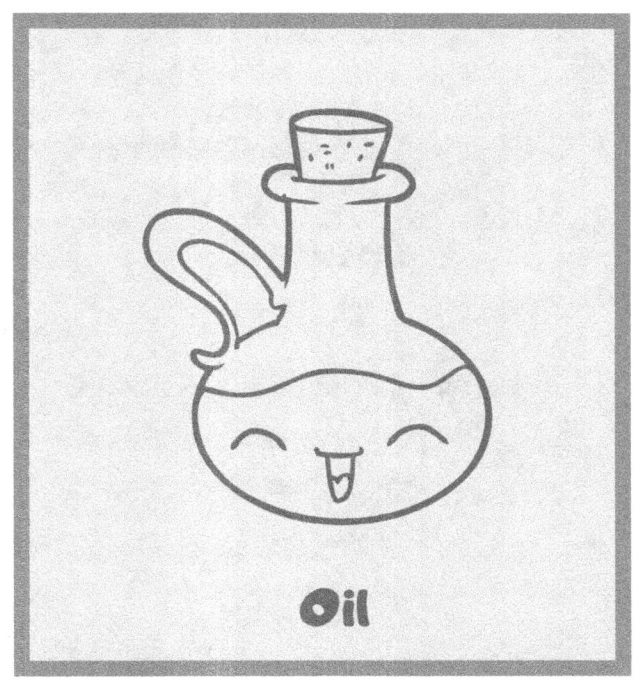

Oil

Fats include oil, mayonnaise, salad dressings, and butter.

They help us feel full, feed all of your cells and make you feel better!

My favorite fat is:

_____

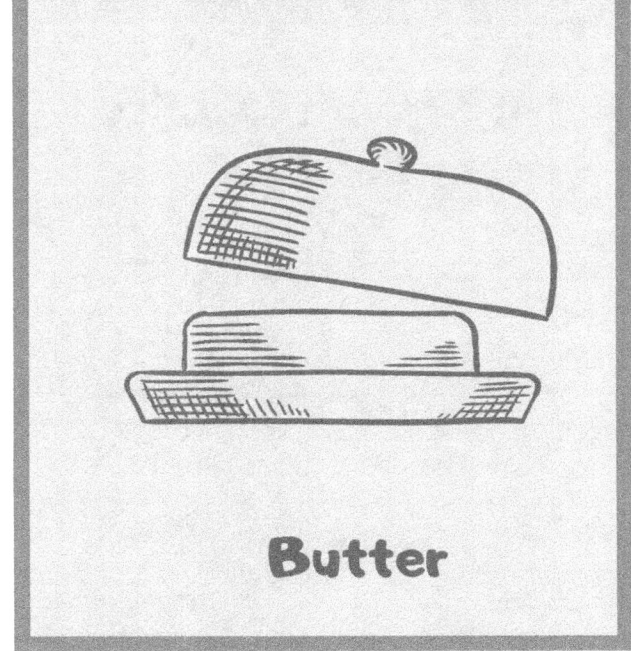

Butter

DAIRY

discover, learn & enjoy delicious dairy foods

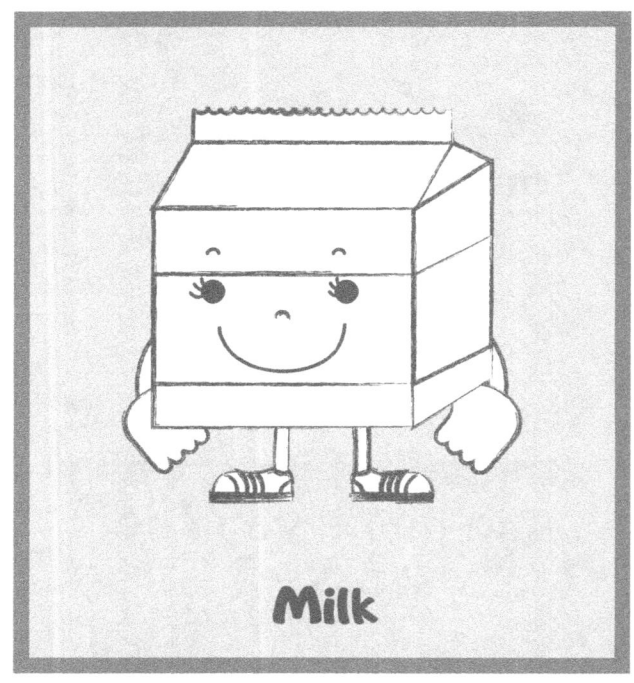

Milk

Dairy foods include milk and all kinds of cheese.

They give us strong bones from our heads to our toes, even your knees!

My favorite dairy food is:

_____

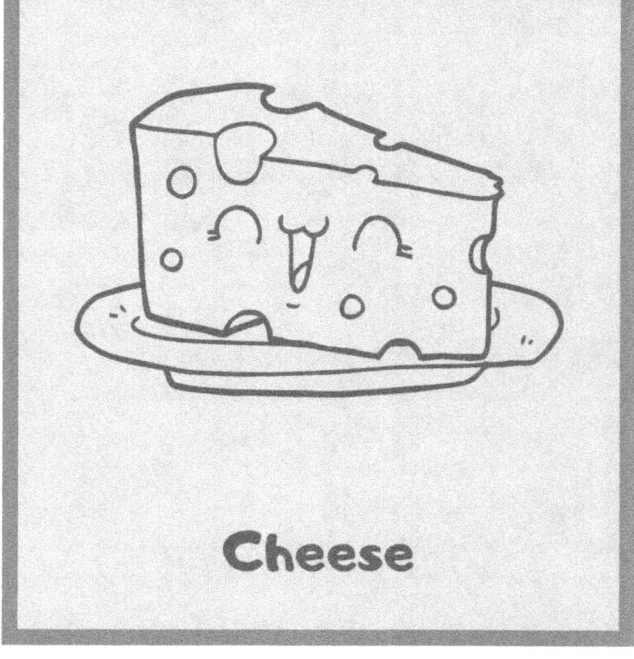

Cheese

FUN FRUIT
COLORING

DAIRY
COLORING

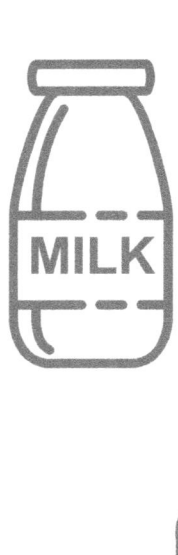

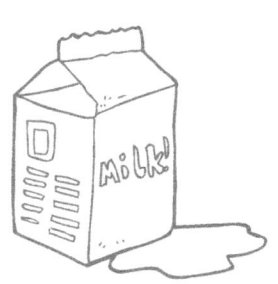
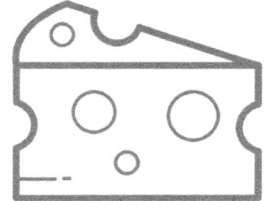
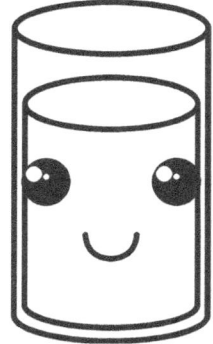

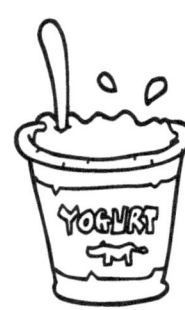
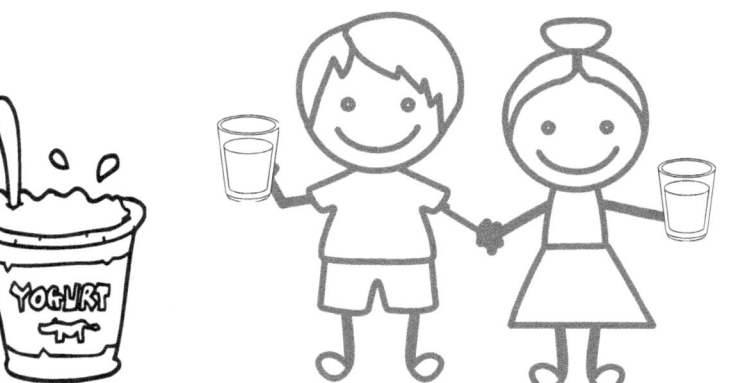

GRAINS
COLORING

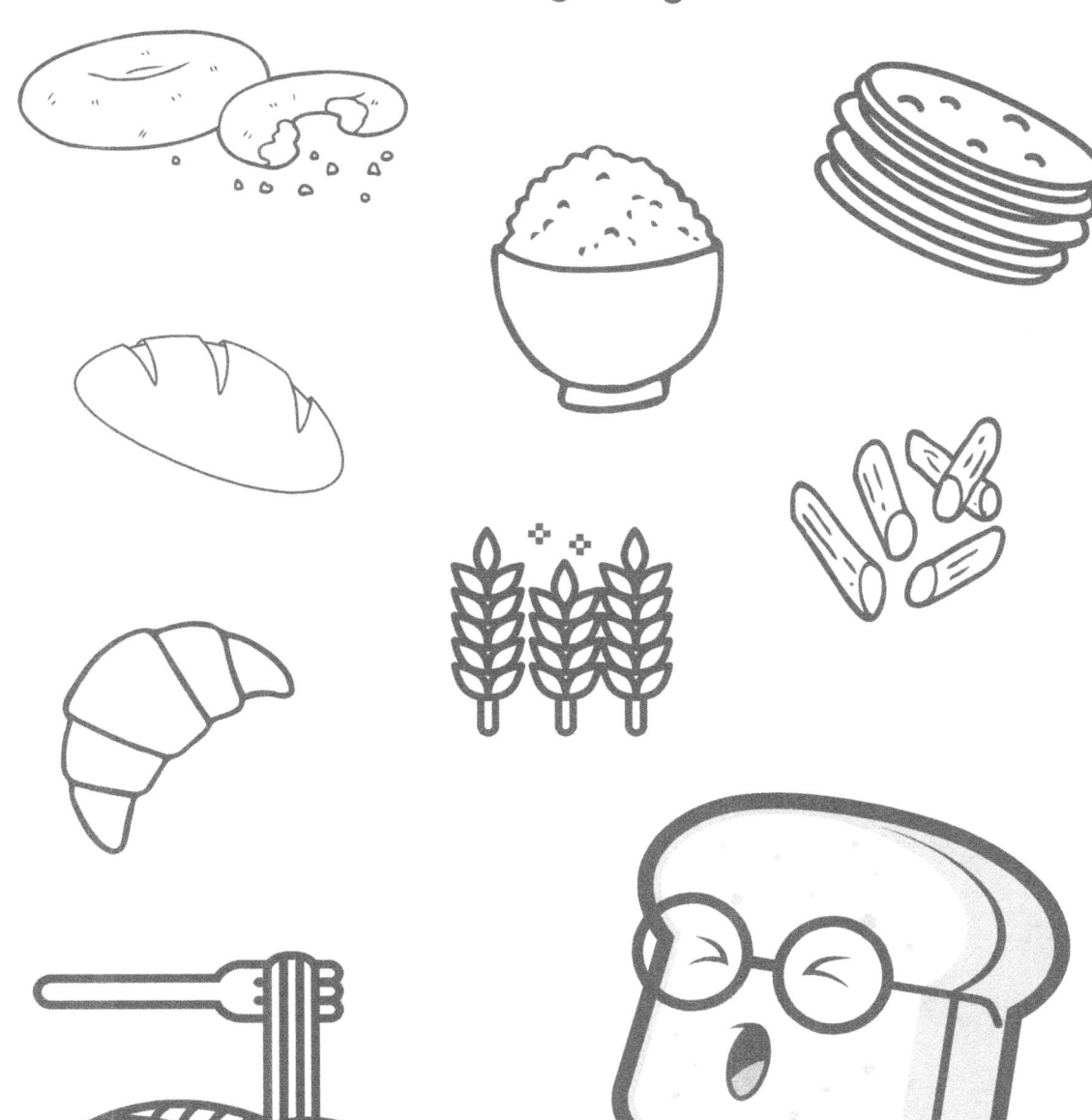

VEGETABLE
COLORING

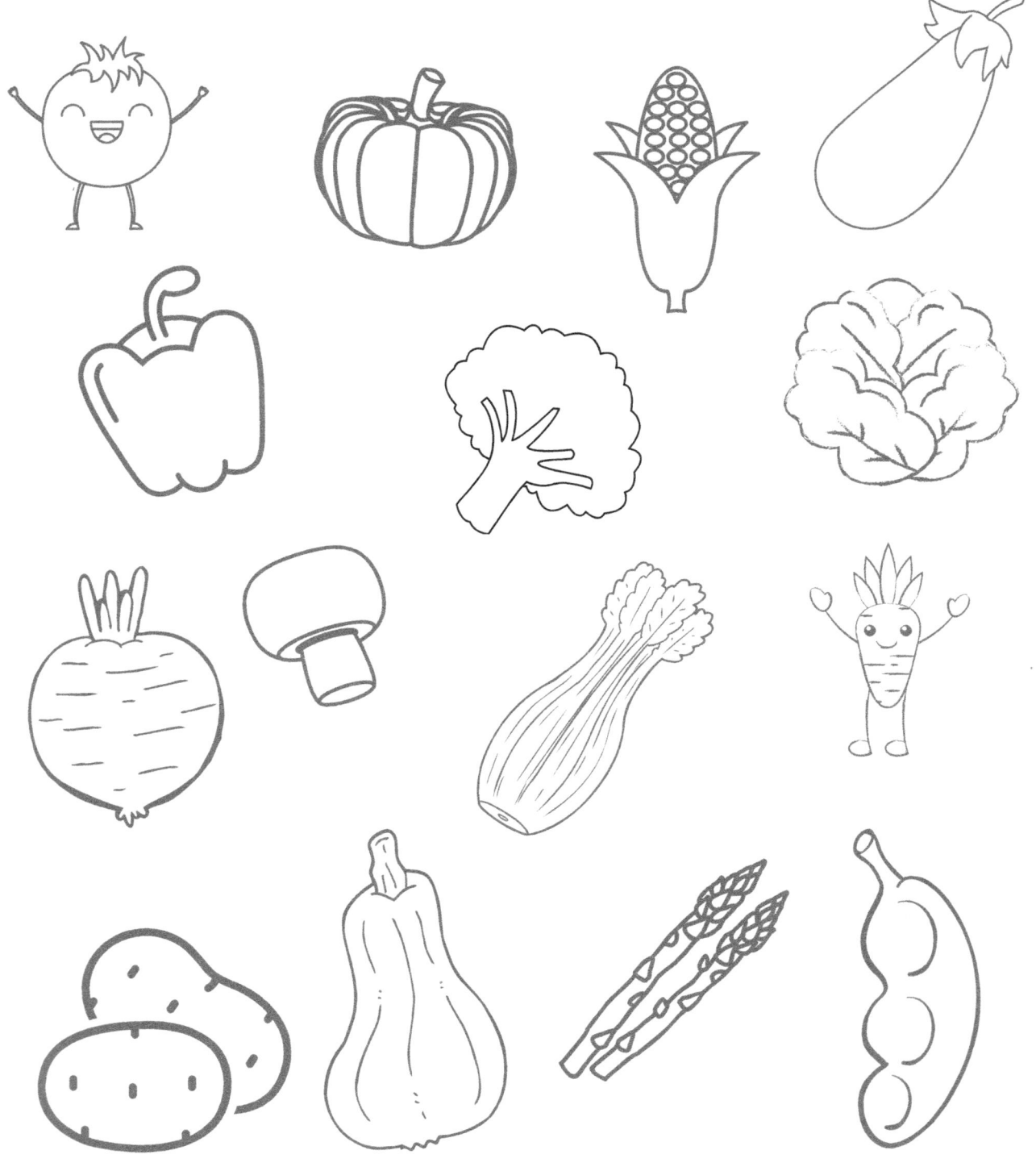

PROTEIN

COLORING

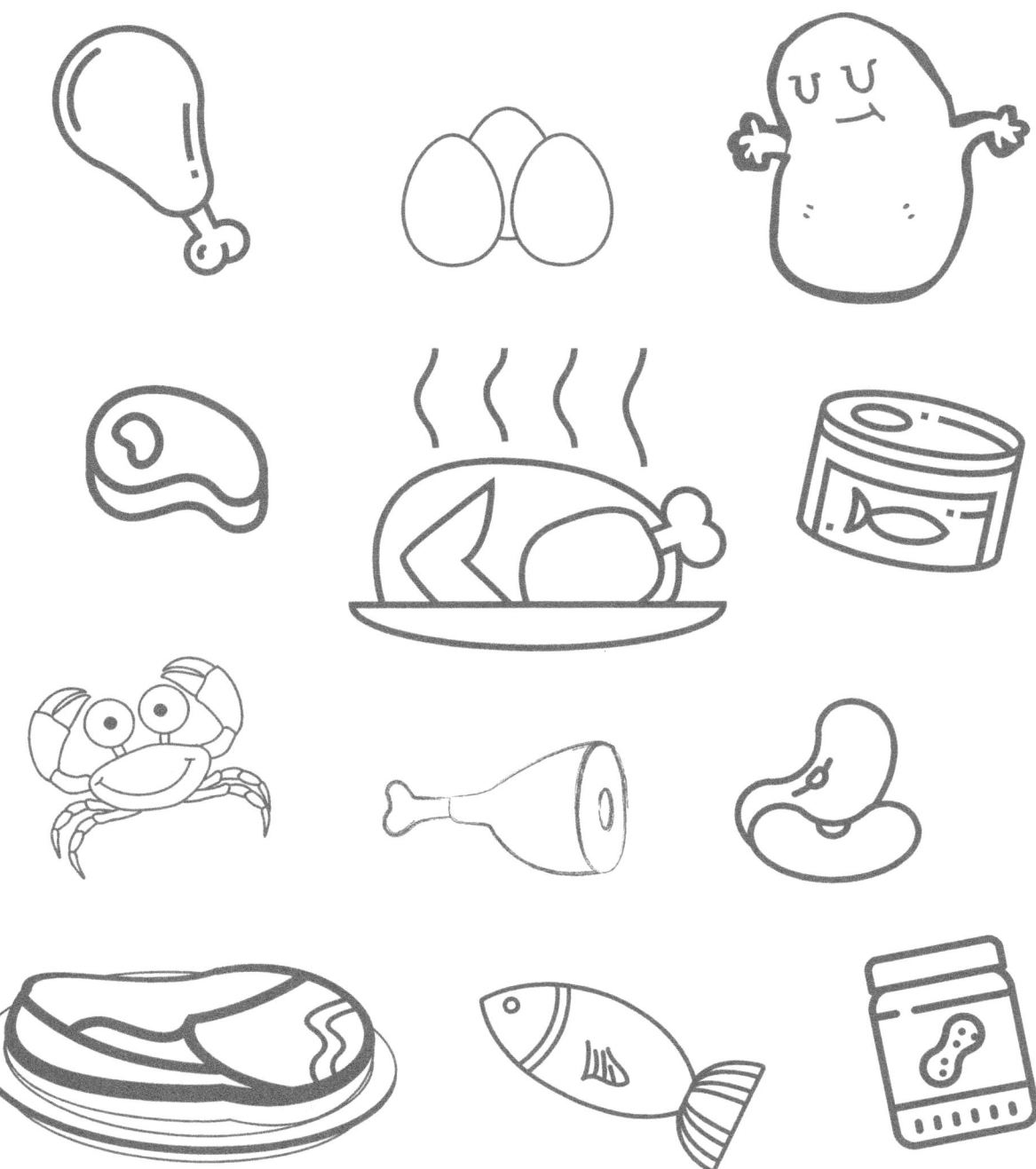

FATS

COLORING

Name: _____

DIRECTIONS: TRACE THE WORDS THAT BEGIN WITH THE LETTER A

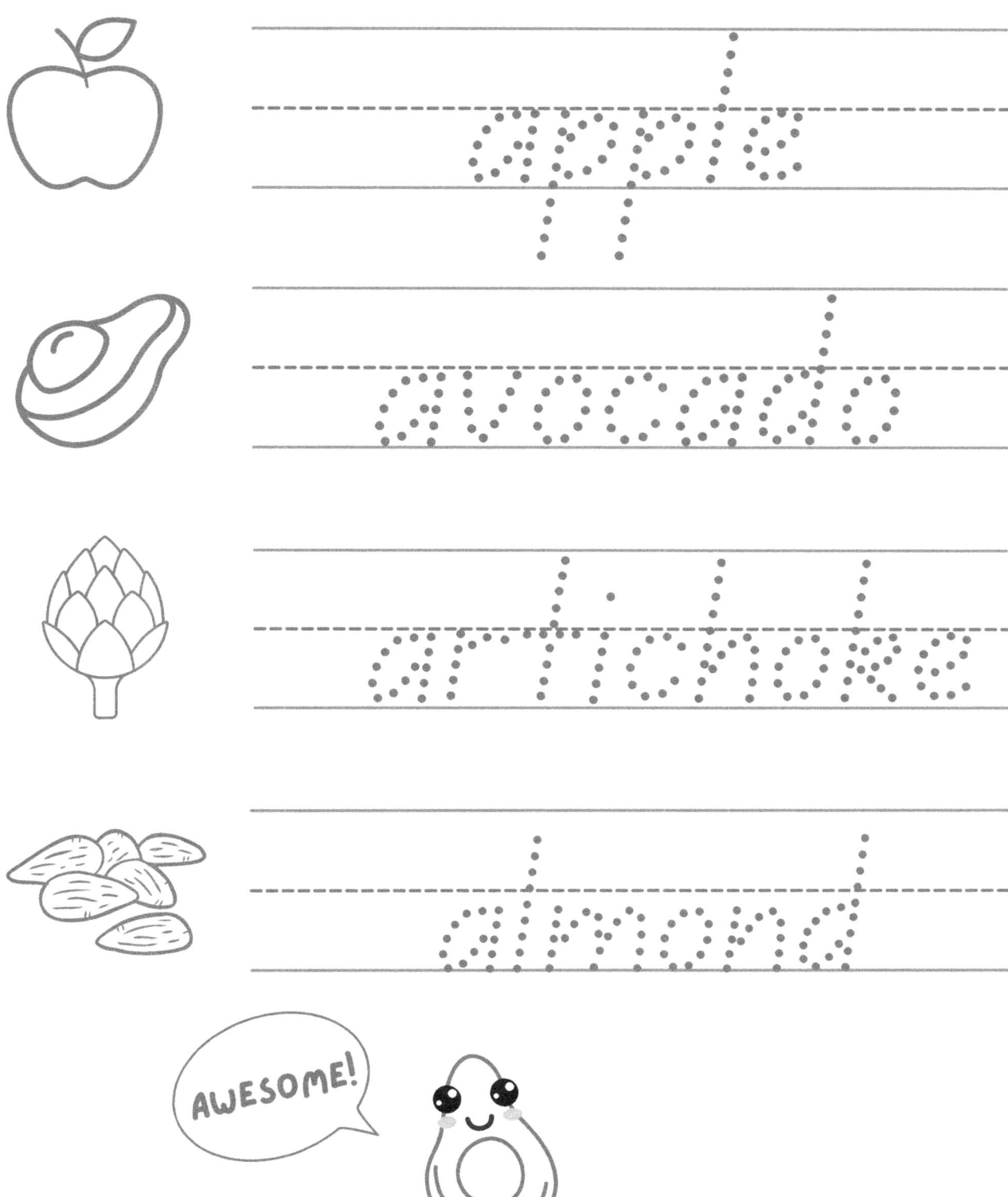

apple

avocado

artichoke

almond

AWESOME!

Is it More or Less?

Learn the concept of more and less.

Instructions: Color the fruits in the right column. If there are more fruits in the right column than in the left, color them red. If there are less fruits in the right column then in the left, color them blue.

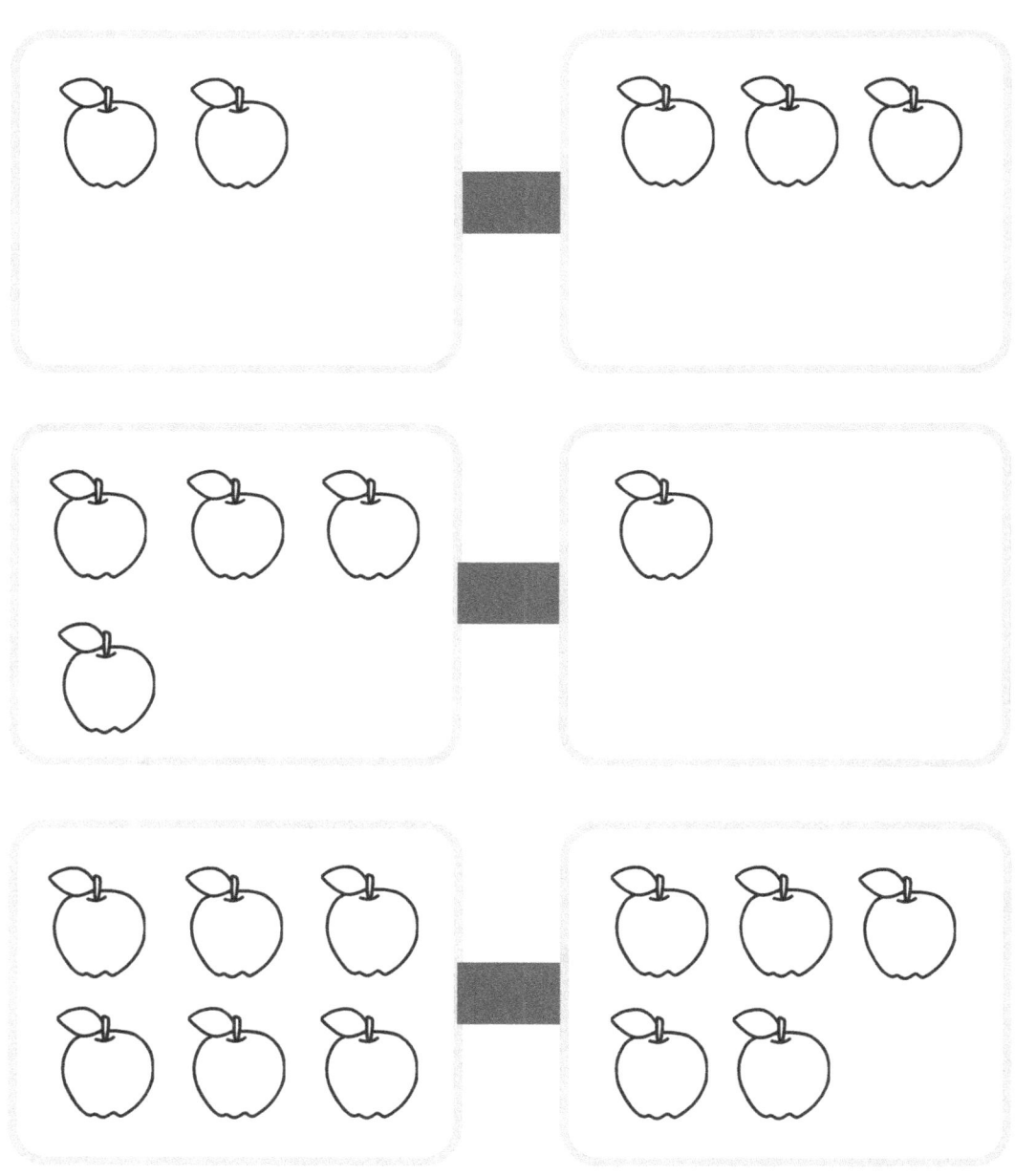

Name: _____   Date: _____

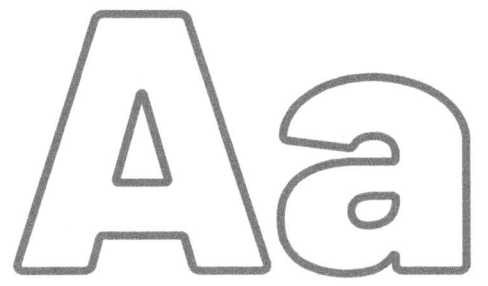 A is for Apple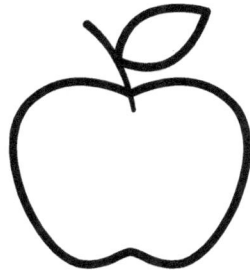

Color the objects that begin with the letter A

   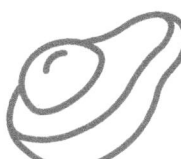      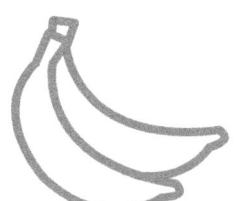

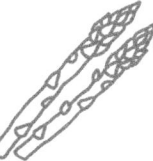         

Trace the letter A and continue writing on the second line

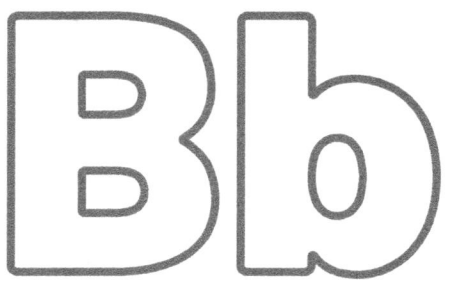 **B is for Broccoli**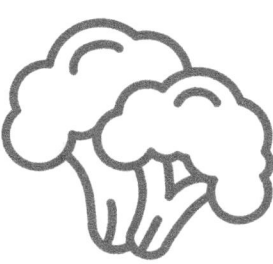

Color the objects that begin with the letter B

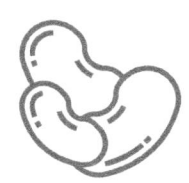 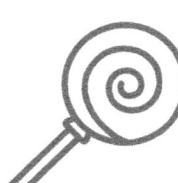 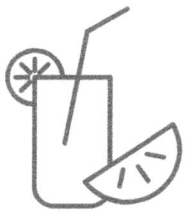 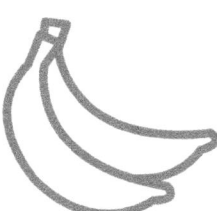

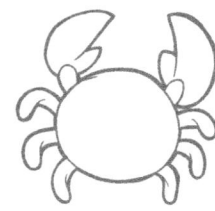 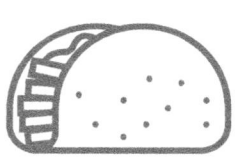 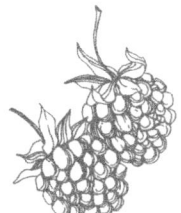 

Trace the letter B and continue writing on the second line

B B B B B

Name: _____ Date: _____

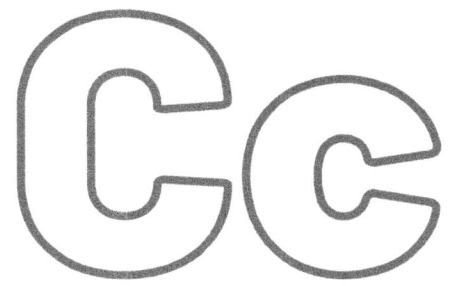 C is for Carrot

Color the objects that begin with the letter C

 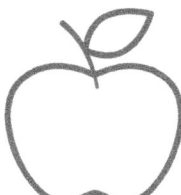 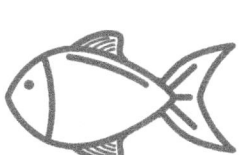 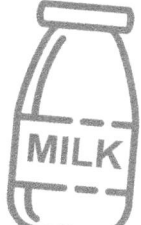

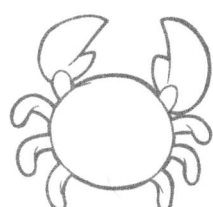 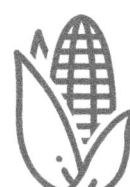 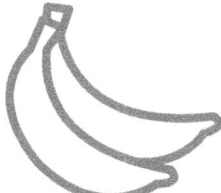 

Trace the letter C and continue writing on the second line

C C C C C C

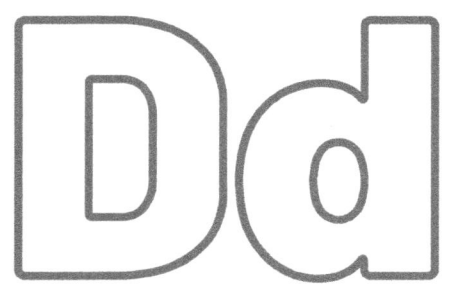 D is for Donut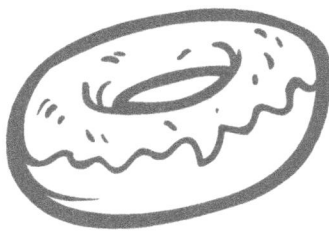

Color the objects that begin with the letter D

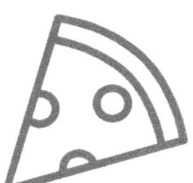  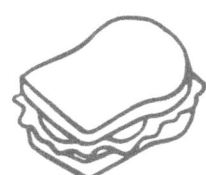 

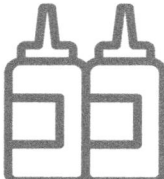 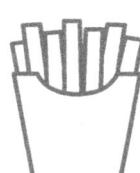 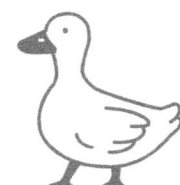 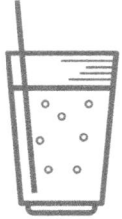

Trace the letter D and continue writing on the second line

Name: _____   Date: _____

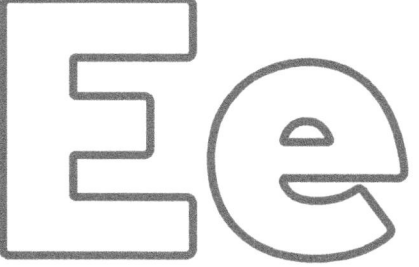 E is for Eggs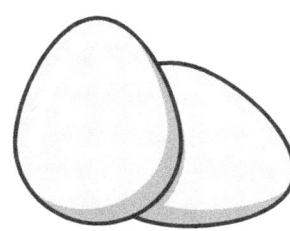

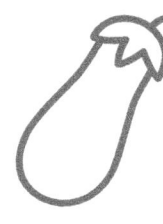 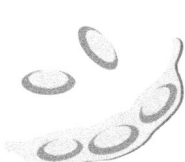 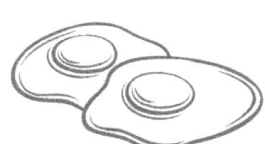 

  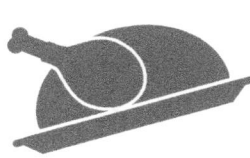 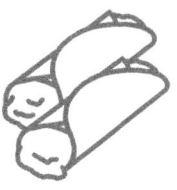

Trace the letter E and continue writing on the second line

Name: _____   Date: _____

Ff

F is for Fish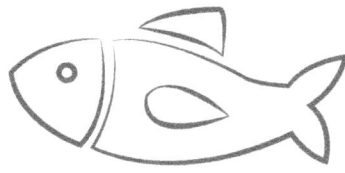

Color the objects that begin with the letter F

 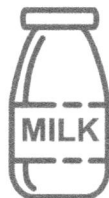 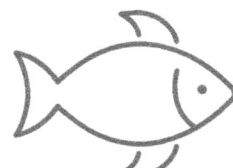 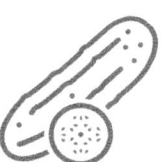

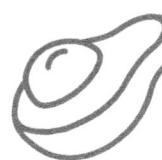 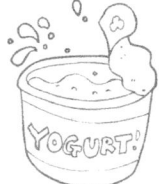  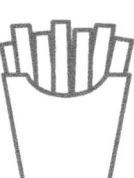

Trace the letter F and continue writing on the second line

Name: _____   Date: _____

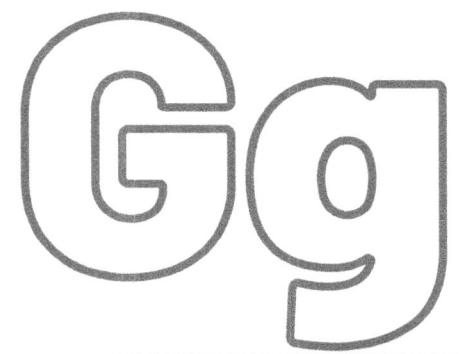 G is for Grapes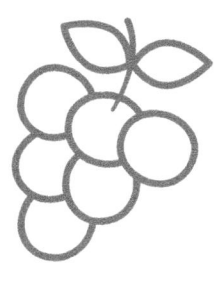

Color the objects that begin with the letter G

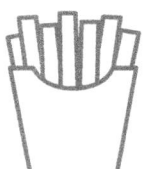   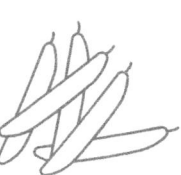

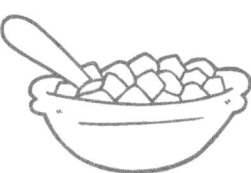   

Trace the letter G and continue writing on the second line

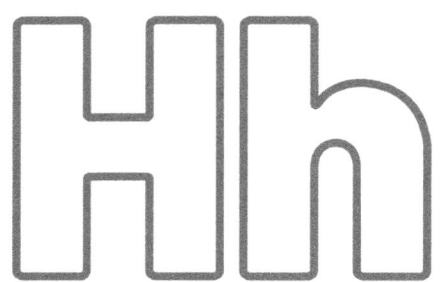 H is for Hotdog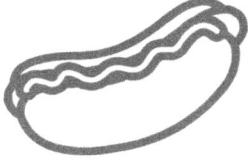

Color the objects that begin with the letter H

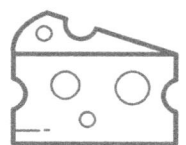 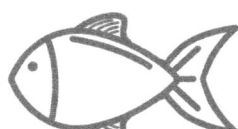 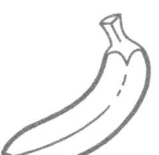 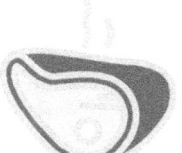

  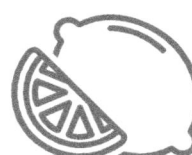 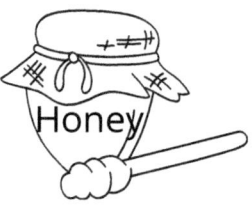

Trace the letter H and continue writing on the second line

Name: _____   Date: _____

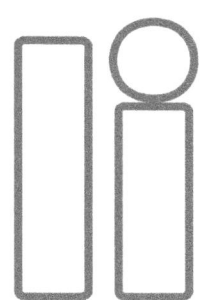   I is for Ice Cream

Color the objects that contain the letter I

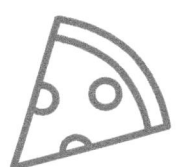   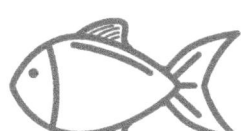   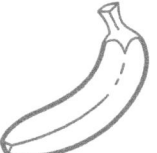   

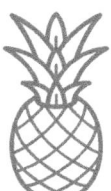   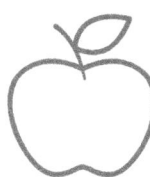      

Trace the letter I and continue writing on the second line

Name: _____   Date: _____

Jj

J is for Jam

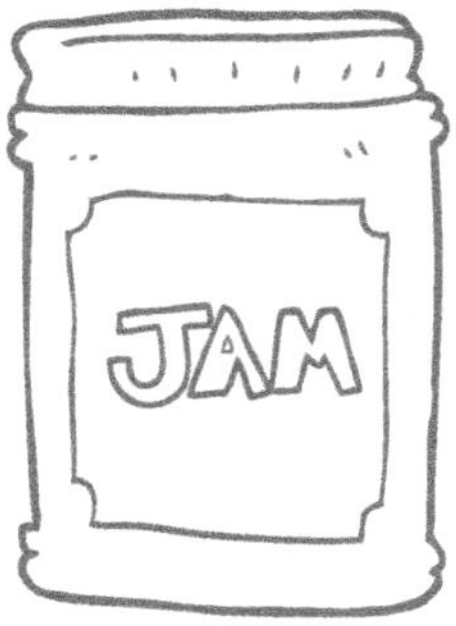

Color the objects that begin with the letter J

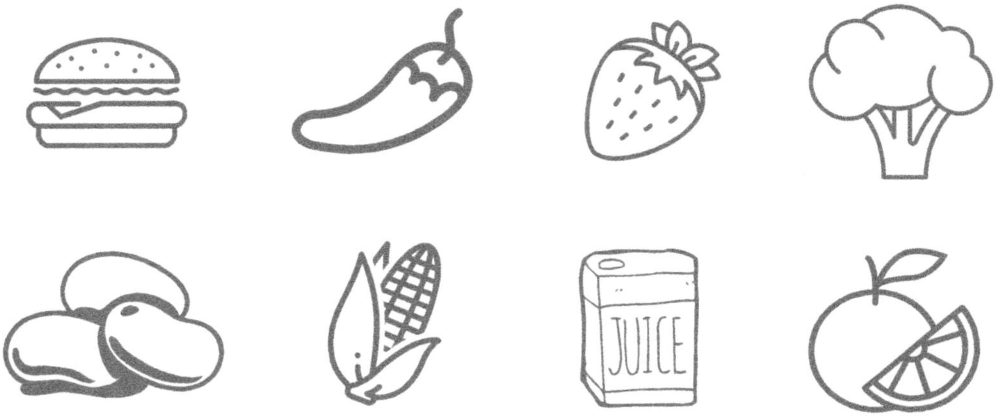

Trace the letter J and continue writing on the second line

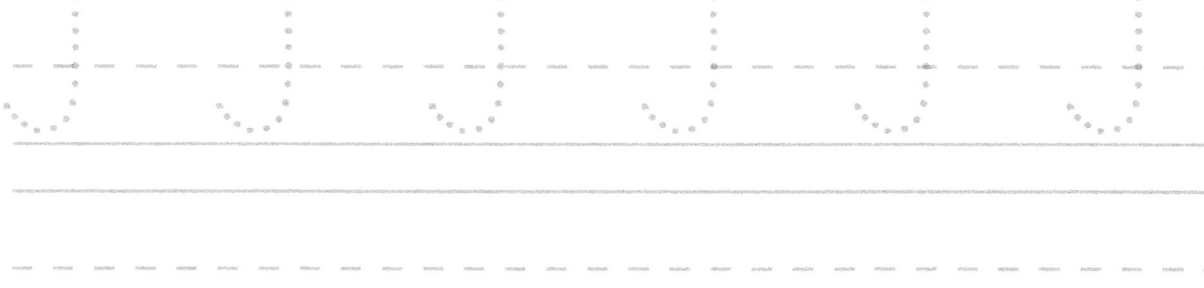

Kk

K is for Kiwi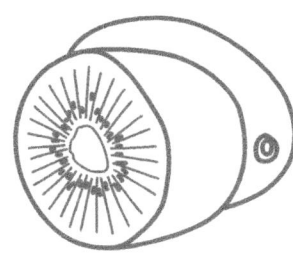

Color the objects that begin with the letter K

  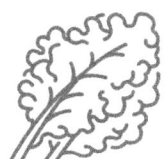 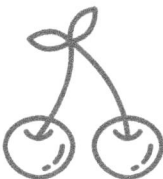

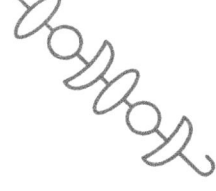  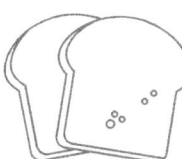 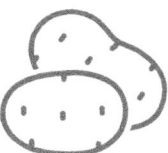

Trace the letter K and continue writing on the second line

K KK K K K K

Name: _____   Date: _____

Ll

L is for Lemon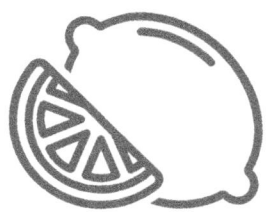

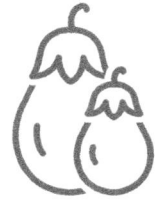  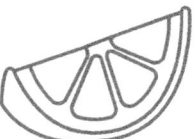 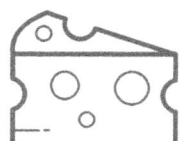

 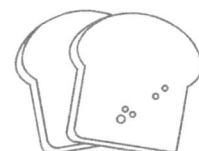 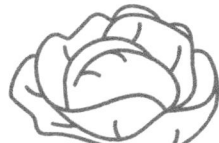 

Trace the letter L and continue writing on the second line

Name: _____   Date: _____

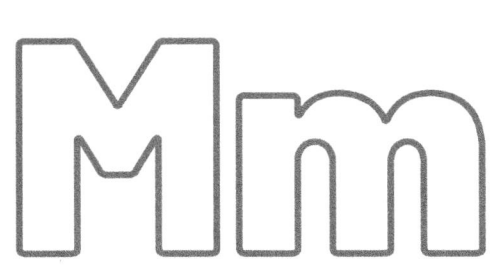 M is for Milk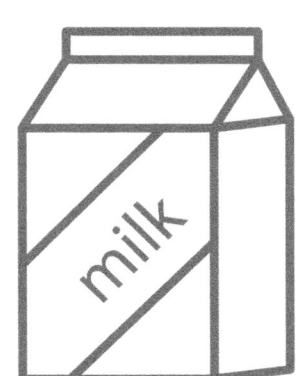

Color the objects that begin with the letter M

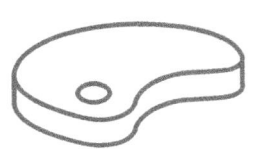  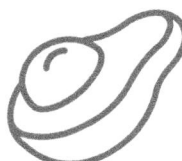 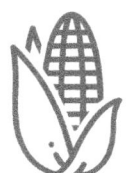

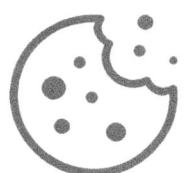 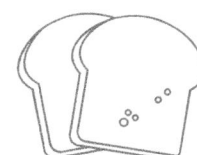 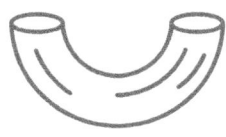 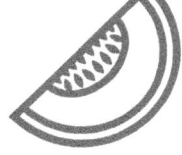

MACARONI

Trace the letter M and continue writing on the second line

M M M M M M

Name: _____   Date: _____

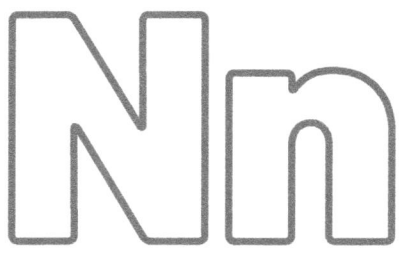 N is for Nuts

Color the objects that begin with the letter N

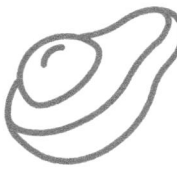  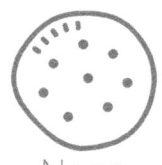 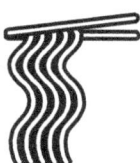

Naan

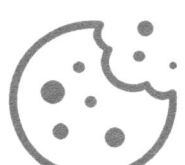 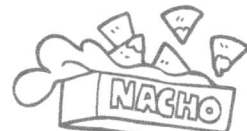  

NACHO

Trace the letter N and continue writing on the second line

N N N N N N

Name: _____   Date: _____

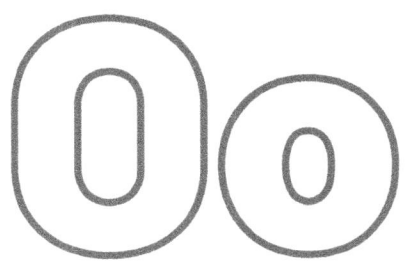 O is for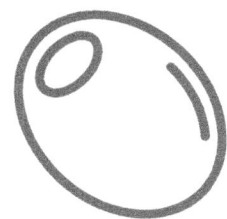

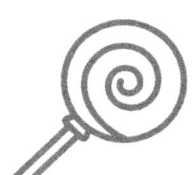 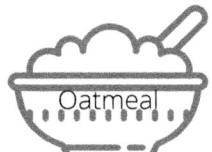 Oatmeal

 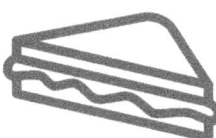 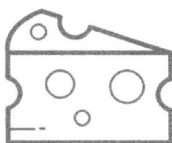 

Trace the letter O and continue writing on the second line

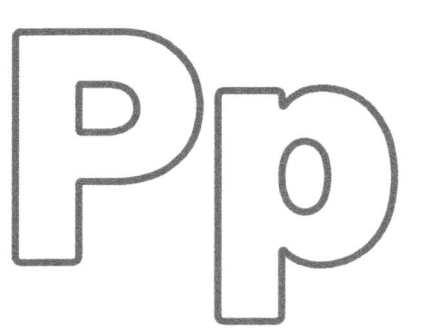

P is for

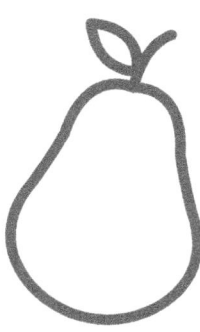

Color the objects that begin with the letter P

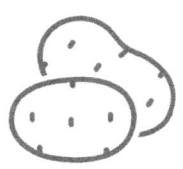
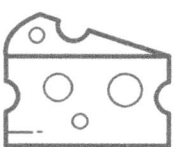
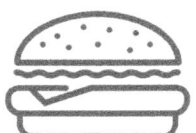
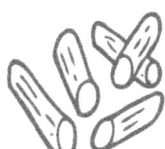

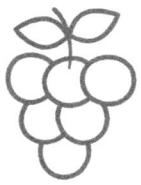
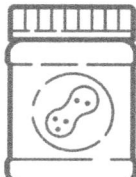

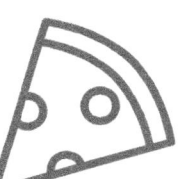

Trace the letter P and continue writing on the second line

Name: _____   Date: _____

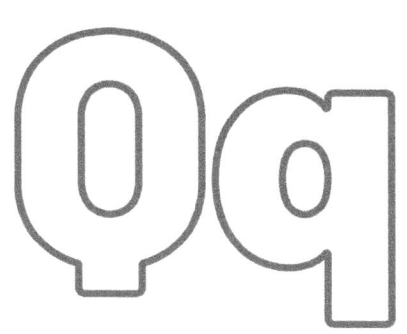 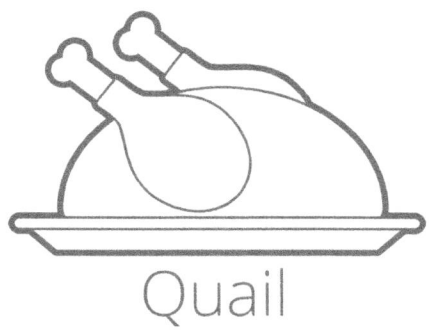

Q is for

Quail

Color the objects that begin with the letter Q

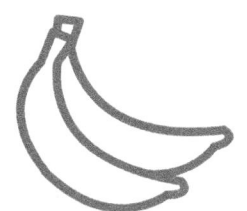 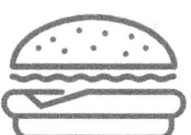 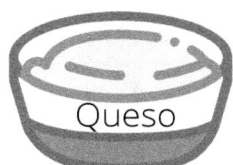

Queso

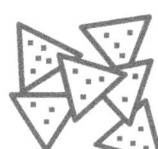

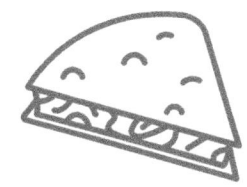  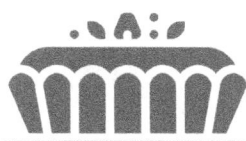 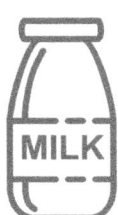

MILK

Trace the letter Q and continue writing on the second line

Name: _____   Date: _____

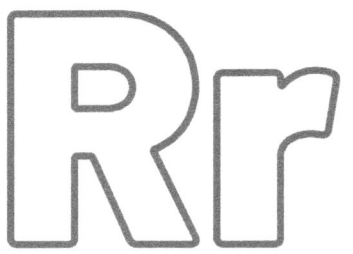 R is for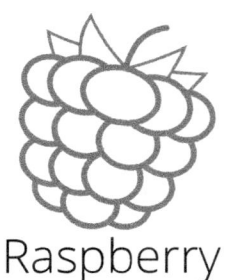
Raspberry

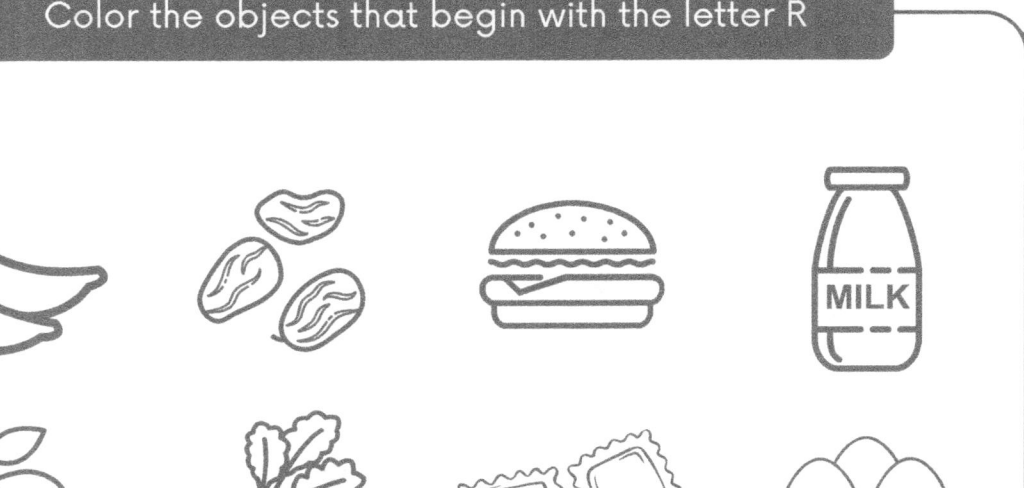

Trace the letter R and continue writing on the second line

Name: _____   Date: _____

S s

S is for

Color the objects that begin with the letter S

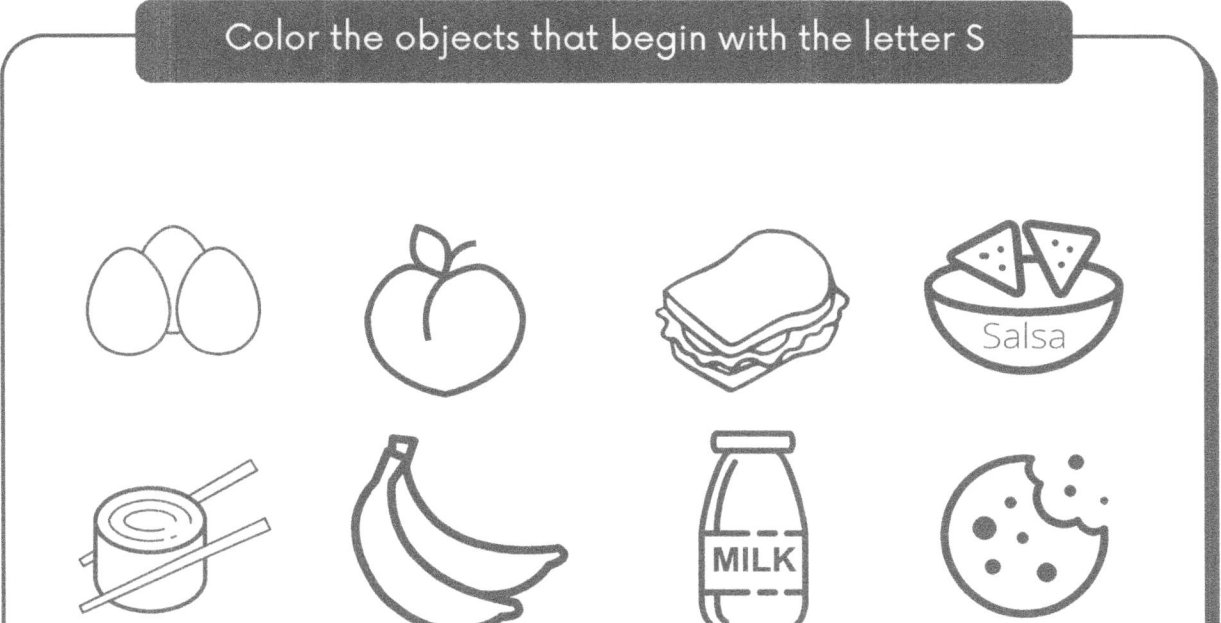

Salsa

MILK

Trace the letter S and continue writing on the second line

S S S S S S

Name: _____   Date: _____

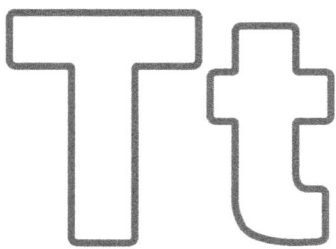 T is for

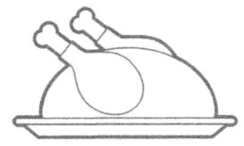   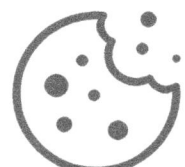

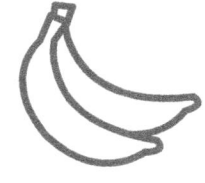 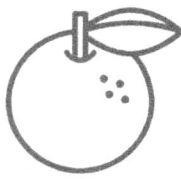 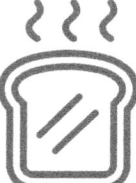 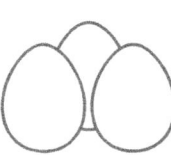

Trace the letter T and continue writing on the second line

Name: _____   Date: _____

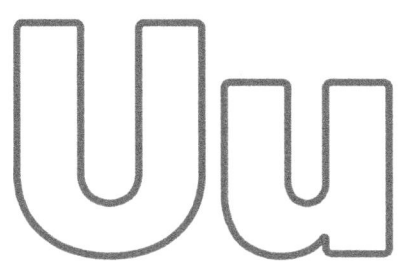 U is for  H(U)ngry

 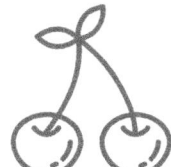 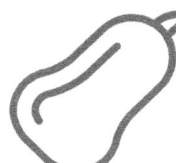 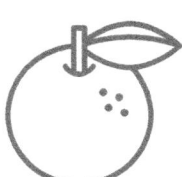

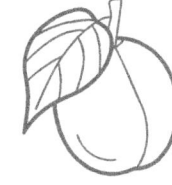 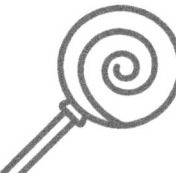 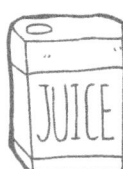 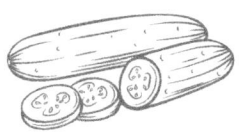

Trace the letter U and continue writing on the second line

V v

V is for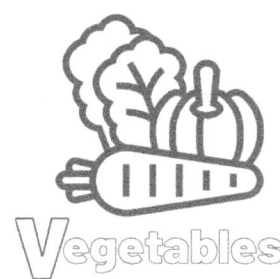
Vegetables

Color the objects that are vegetables

Trace the letter V and continue writing on the second line

Name: _____   Date: _____

Ww W is for

         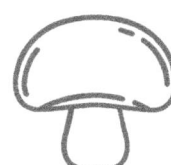

Wasabi

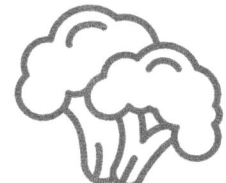      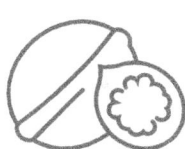   

Trace the letter W and continue writing on the second line

Name: _____   Date: _____

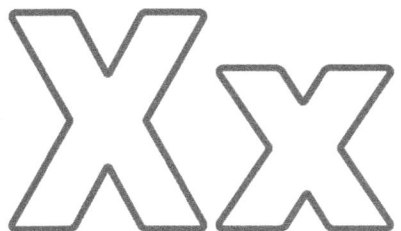 X is for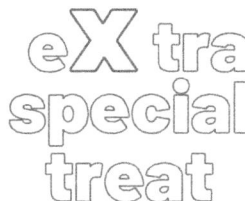

Color the objects that are eXtra special treats!

Trace the letter X and continue writing on the second line

X X X X X

Name: _____   Date: _____

Yy

Y is for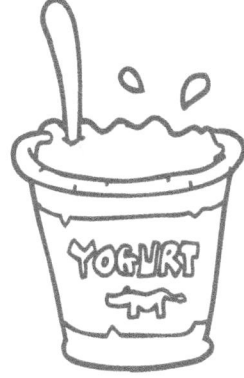

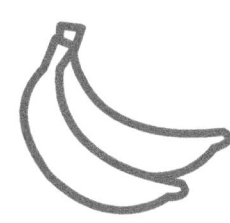 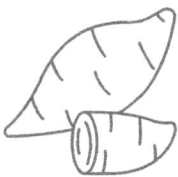 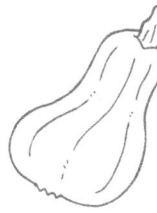 

 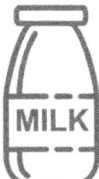  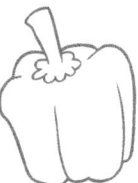

Trace the letter Y and continue writing on the second line

Zz

Z is for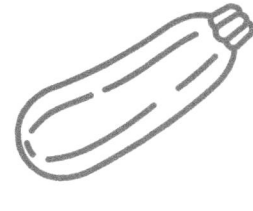

Zucchini

Color the objects that have the letter Z in them

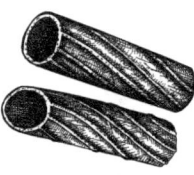
Ziti

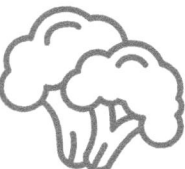

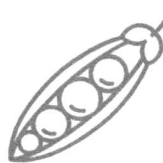

Mozzarella

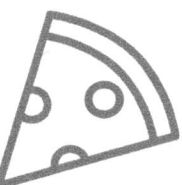

Trace the letter Z and continue writing on the second line

Name: _____

UPPERCASE
HANDWRITING
PRACTICE

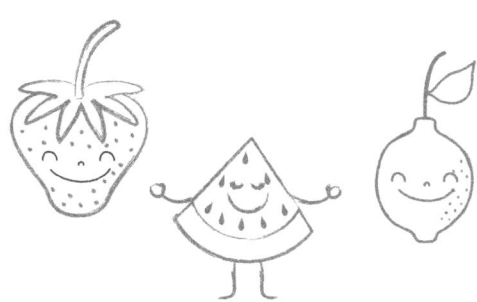

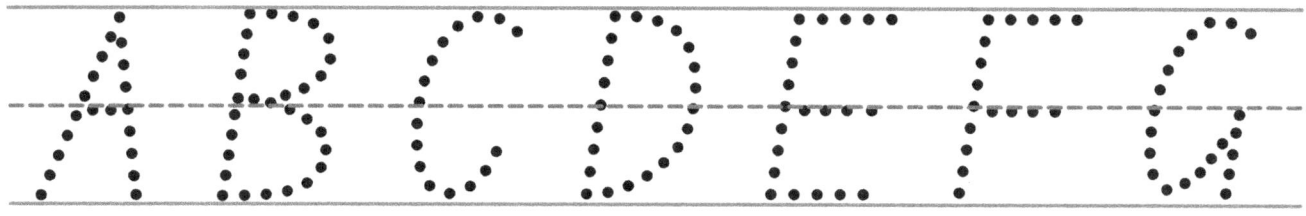

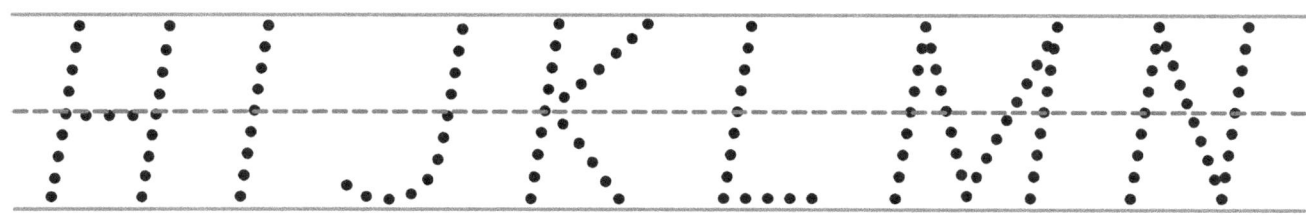

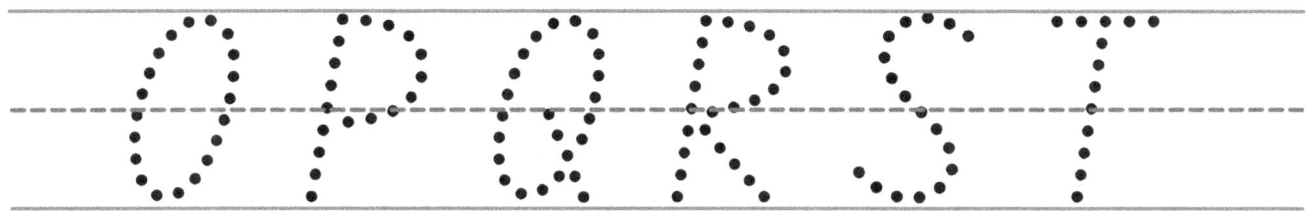

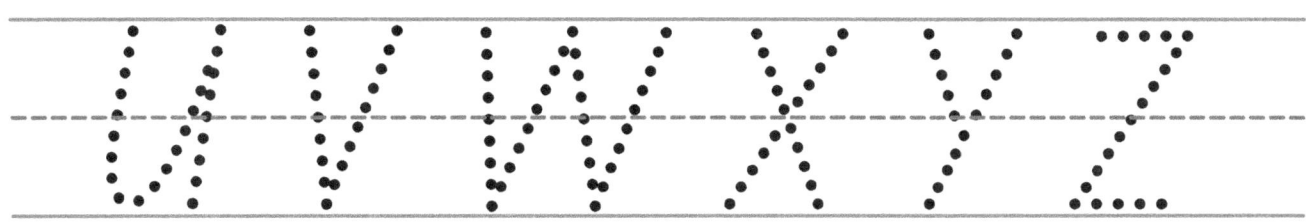

Name: _____

LOWERCASE HANDWRITING PRACTICE

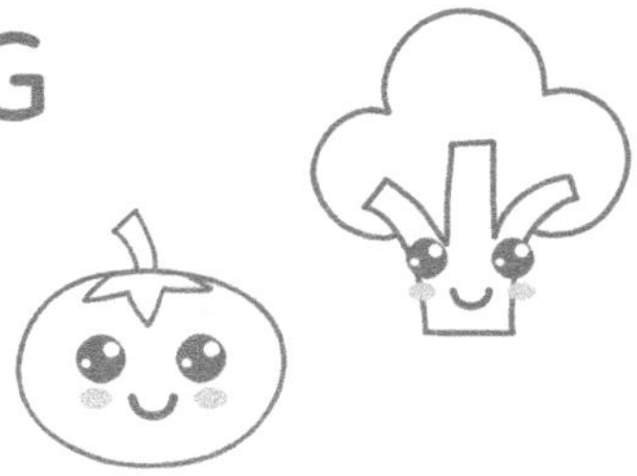

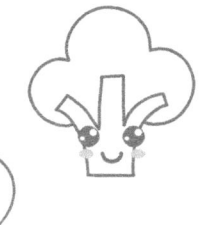

a b c d e f g

h i j k l m n o

p q r s t u v

w x y z

PROTEIN POWER!

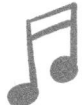

Protein Power!
I've got the Protein Power!
I'm talking breakfast, lunch and dinner or whenever you eat
You need some healthy protein it just can't be beat!

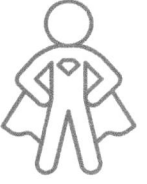

Chicken, meat and fish; nuts and eggs, too
We need some healthy protein for me and for you!
Peanut butter, beans, tofu, and lots of legumes
Are healthy protein choices to give us some zoom!
So eat some protein at each meal, you can't go wrong
Eating protein all day long will make you big and strong!
Protein Power!
I've got the Protein Power!

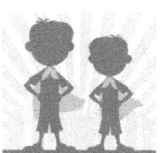

Draw your favorite protein, then draw your favorite superpower!

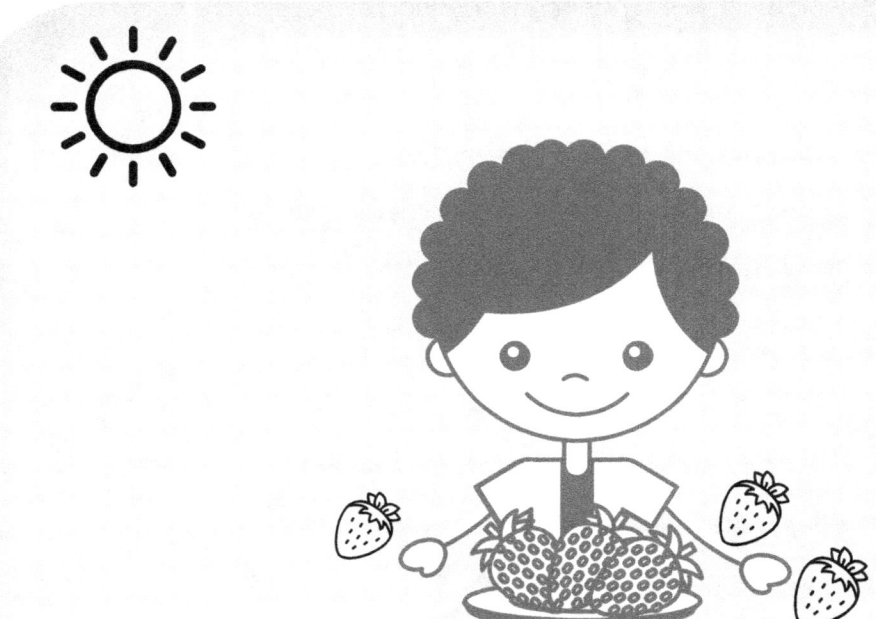

Sam eats strawberries on a sunny day.

Trace the sentence on the lines below.

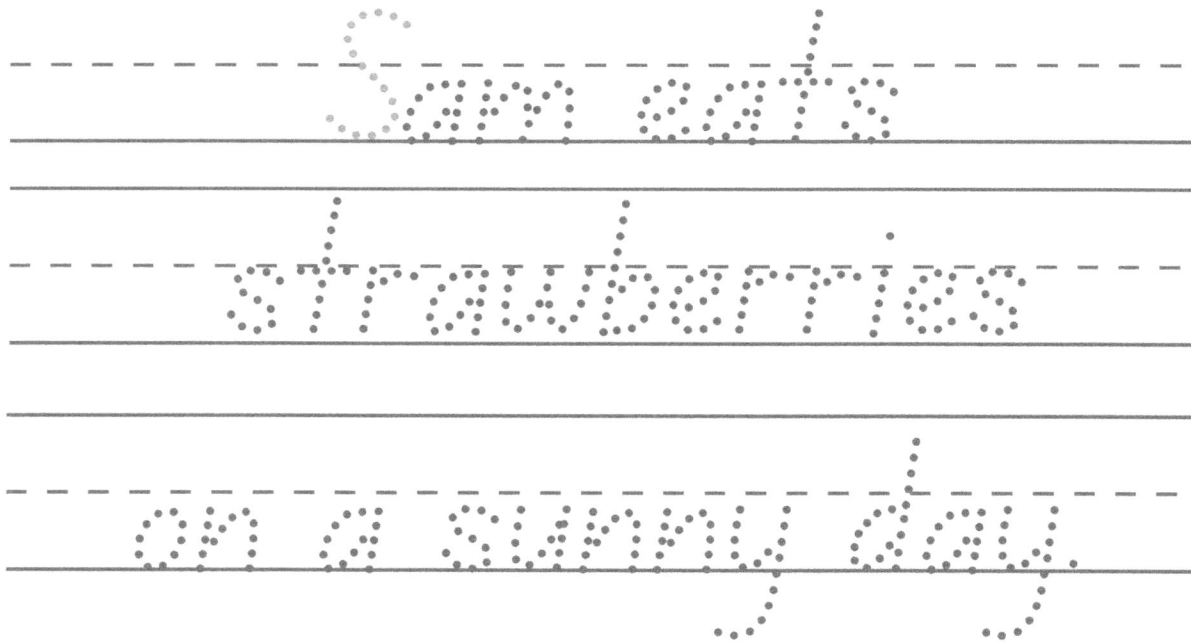

Name: _____

THE FRUIT EXPRESS

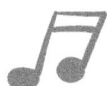
Fruit-a Fruit-a
Fruit-a Fruit-a
Chew Chew! Yummy!
Let's hop aboard the Fruit Express
Tell me about the fruit
that you like best!

Draw a picture of you eating your favorite fruit.

VEGETABLES

PRACTICE WRITING THE FOLLOWING WORDS.

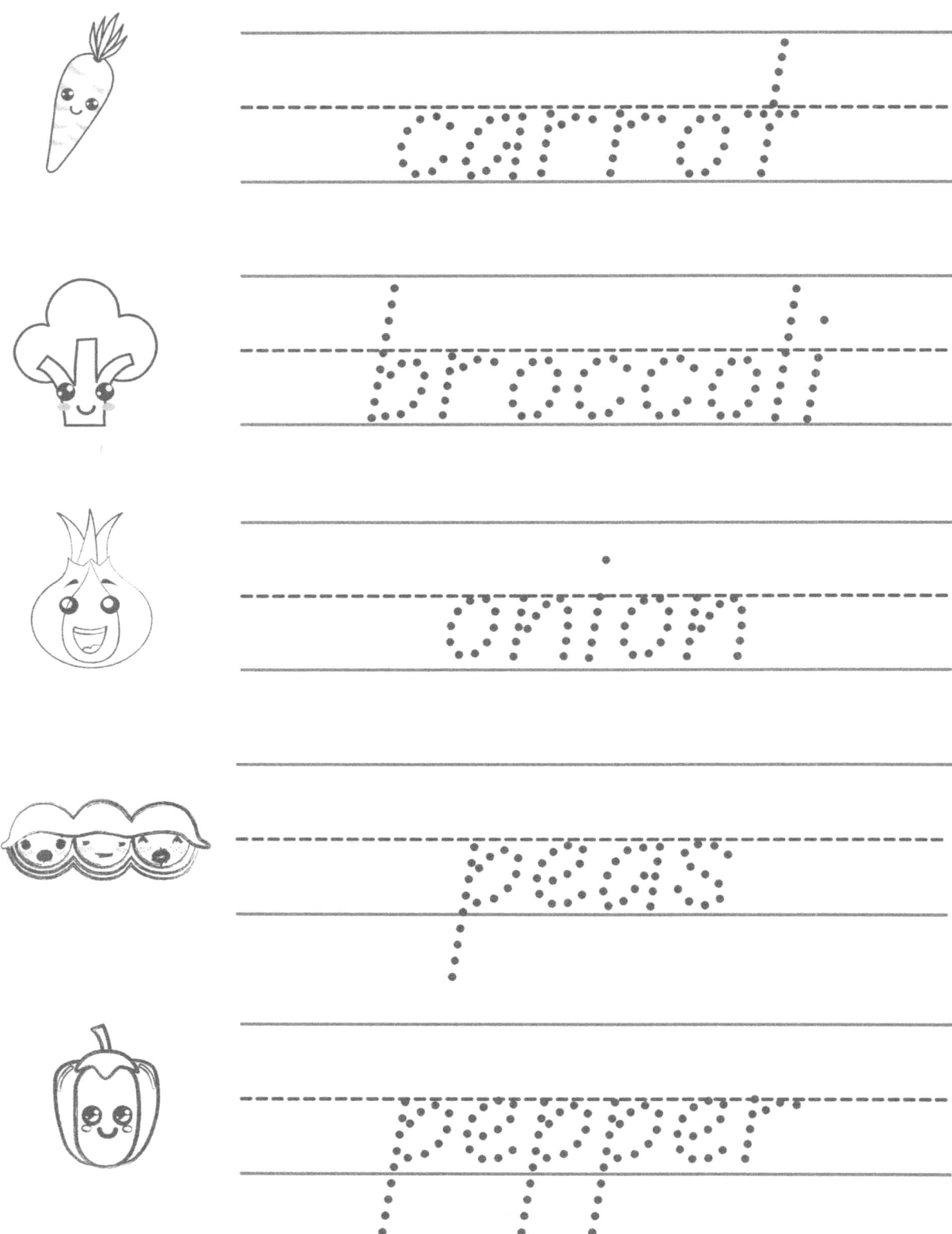

carrot

broccoli

onion

peas

pepper

Name:

DAIRY

PRACTICE WRITING THE FOLLOWING WORDS.

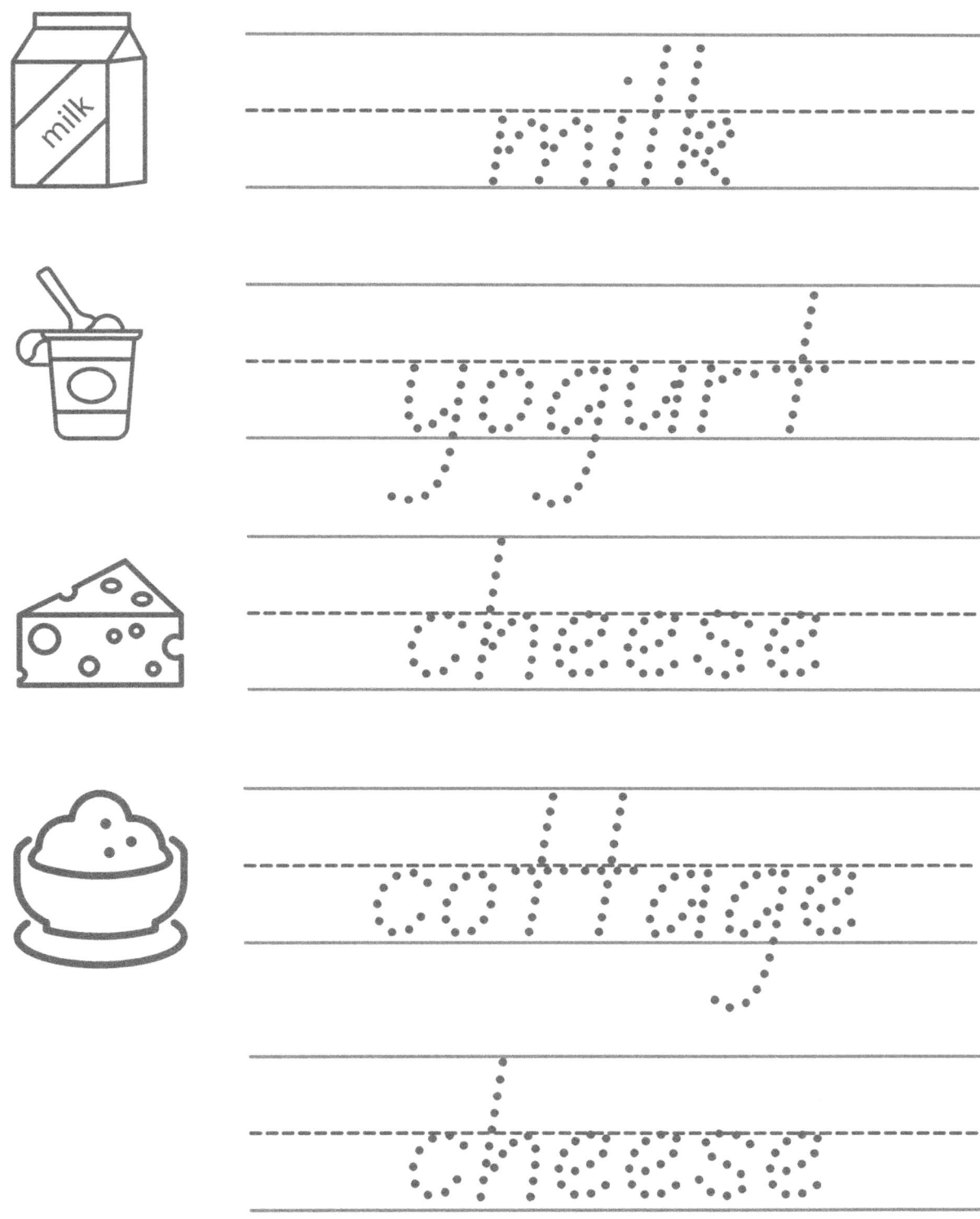

Name: _____

GRAINS

PRACTICE WRITING THE FOLLOWING WORDS.

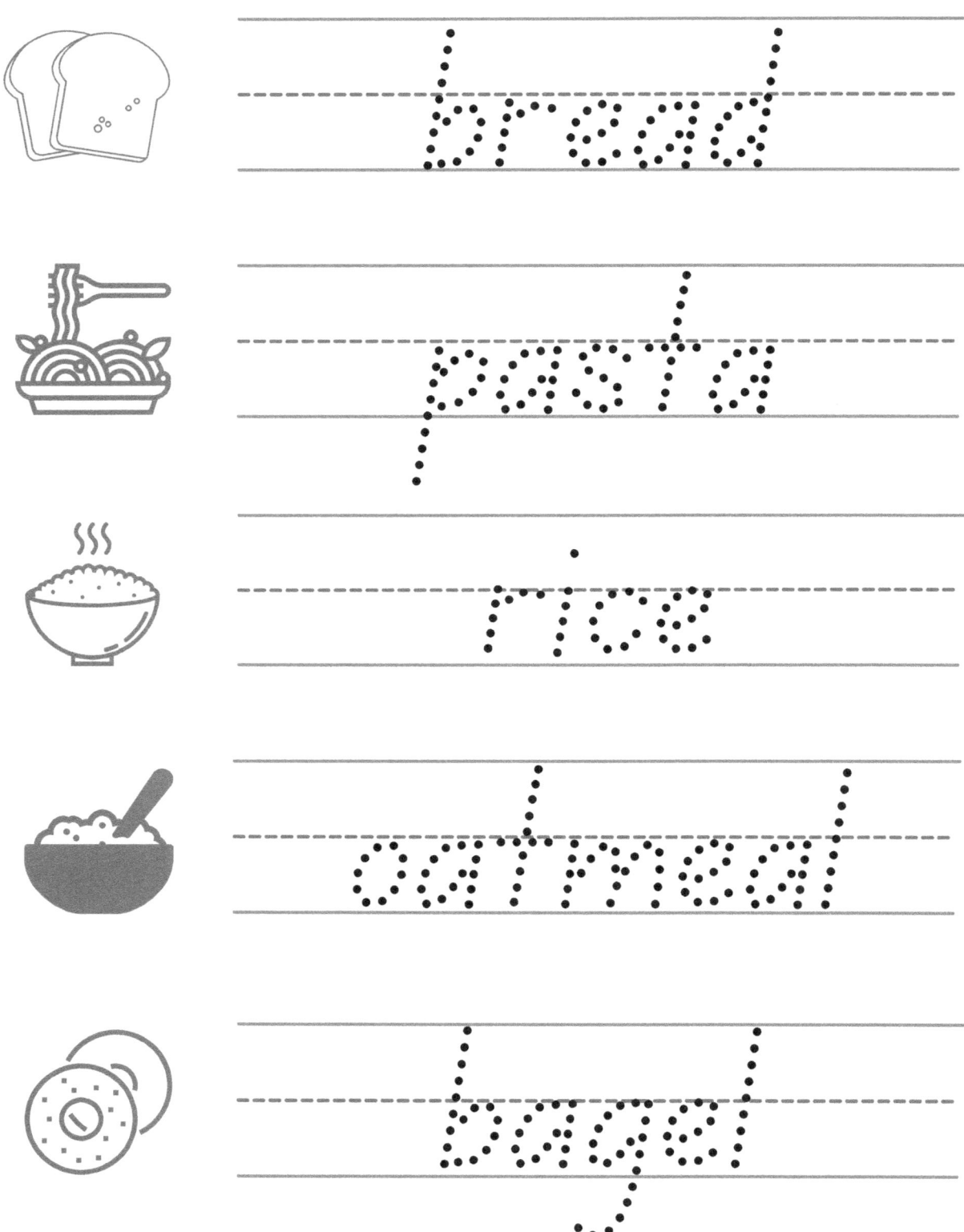

bread

pasta

rice

oatmeal

bagel

PROTEIN

PRACTICE WRITING THE FOLLOWING WORDS.

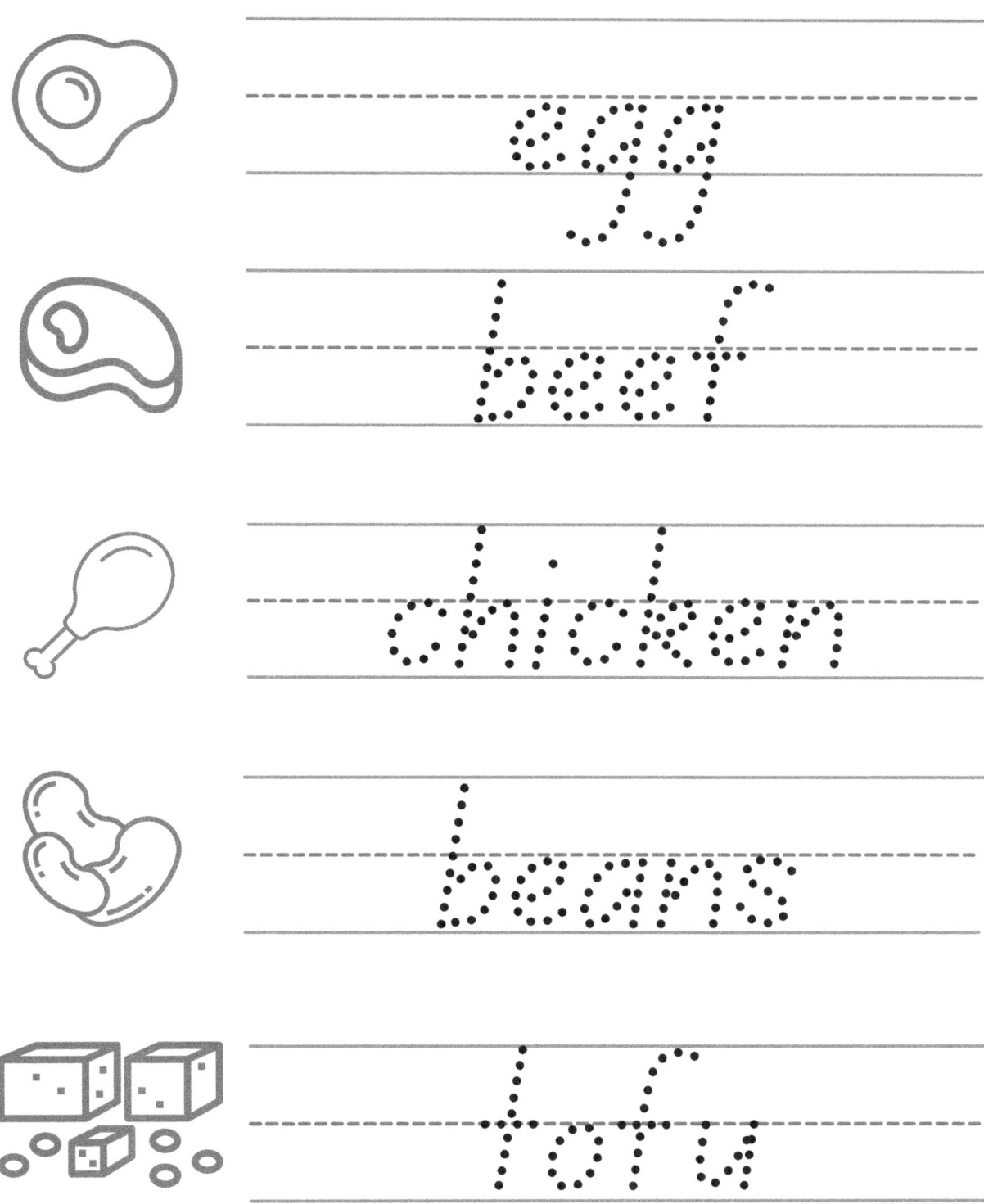

FRUIT

PRACTICE WRITING THE FOLLOWING WORDS.

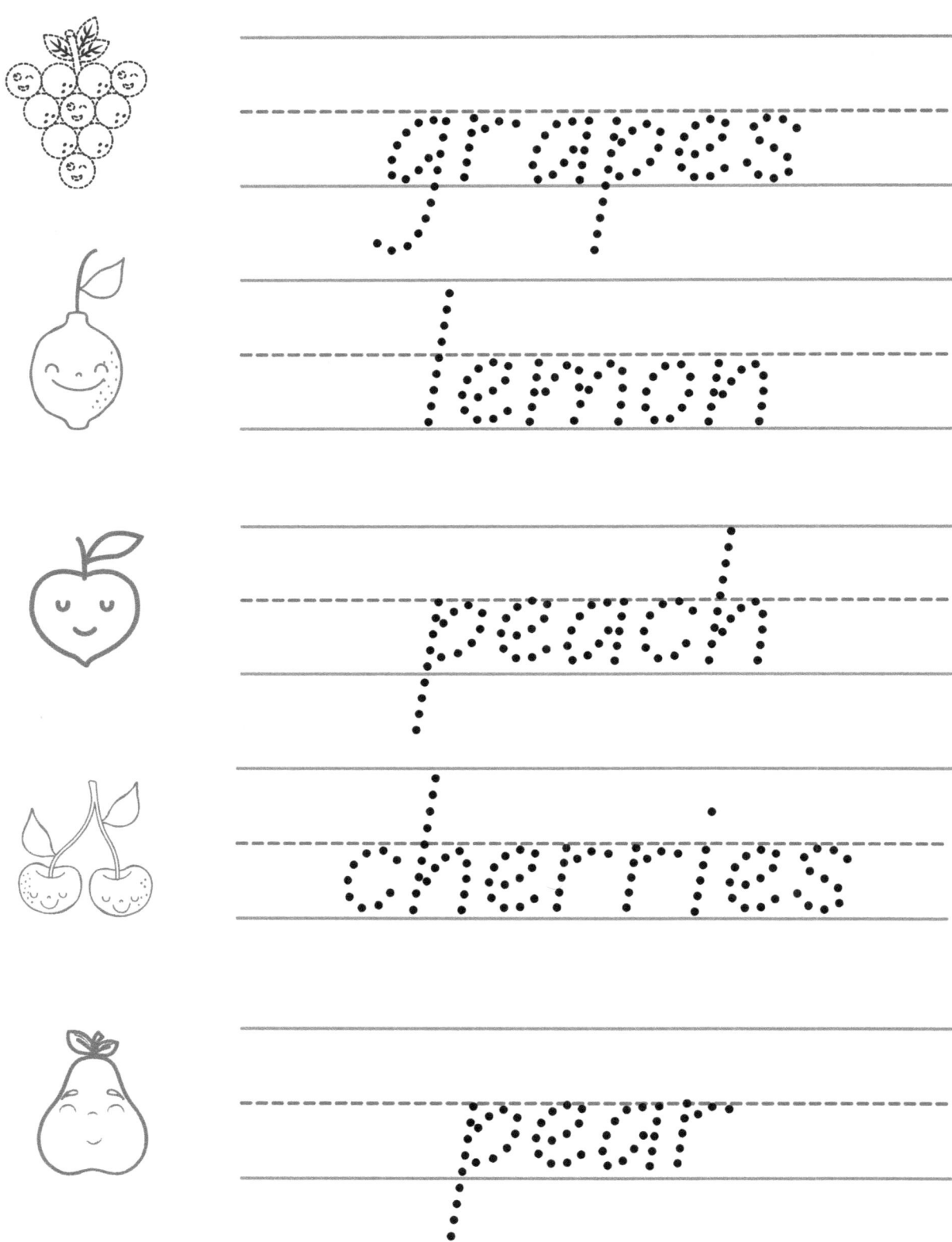

Name: _____

FATS

PRACTICE WRITING THE FOLLOWING WORDS.

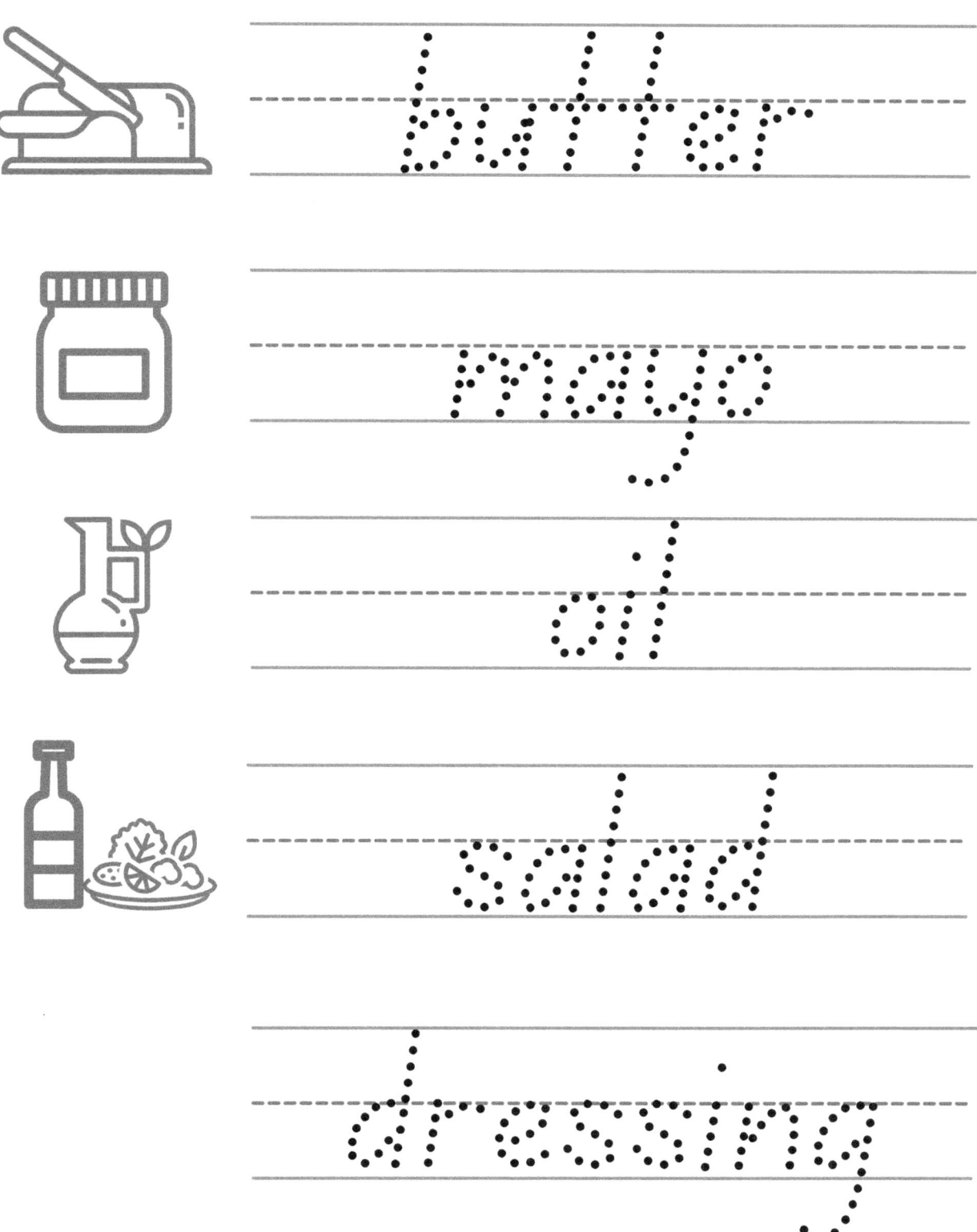

butter

mayo

oil

salad

dressing

Certificate
of
Completion

Presented to:

_____

Name

for successfully completing the
Food is Fun! ABC's workbook.

_____

Date

Way to Go!

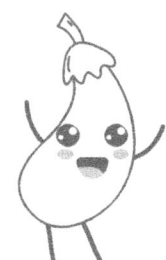